Advance Praise for S

There are no better guides for joy out there than Neal and Carly. As they share their own story with profound simplicity and vulnerability, they highlight a practical approach to emotional wellness. *Start from Joy* is a proven recipe for living a life that matters.

BETH AND JEFF McCORD
Founder of Your Enneagram Coach and authors of *More than Your Number*

In our noble attempts to live purposefully, many of us have forgotten how to experience joy. This biblically based, scientifically sound book provides the antidote. Written by two of the most joyful people I know, *Start from Joy* is a book I highly recommend.

JORDAN RAYNOR
National bestselling author of *Redeeming Your Time*

Like money and happiness, joy is not something to be approached directly. Rather, it is a byproduct of living well. Here's your guide to living in such a way that joy shows up—every day!

DAN MILLER
Author of *48 Days to the Work You Love*

Neal and Carly are two of the most joyful people I've ever met. After reading *Start from Joy*, I finally understand why. Packed with intriguing science, captivating stories, and endless applications, this is the emotional-wellness book written for times like these.

JEFF BROWN
Author of *Read to Lead: The Simple Habit That Expands Your Influence and Boosts Your Career* and host of the *Read to Lead* podcast, a four-time Best Business Podcast nominee

Every week I coach individuals who are stuck, frustrated, and hopeless on the road to positive change. Though I give them the strategies to succeed, there's an invisible barrier that barricades greater achievement and fulfillment in their lives. I couldn't put words to this barrier—that is, until now. *Start from Joy* is the book we all need to read if we want to create lasting positive change in the world.

BRIAN DIXON
Author of *Start with Your People*

What a joy! Neal and Carly have given us a gift in this timely reminder of the power of joy to energize positive change in our lives.

JOSH SPURLOCK, MA, LPC
Founder of MyCounselor.Online

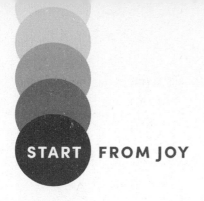

START FROM JOY

NEAL SAMUDRE
CARLY SAMUDRE LPC-MHSP

START FROM

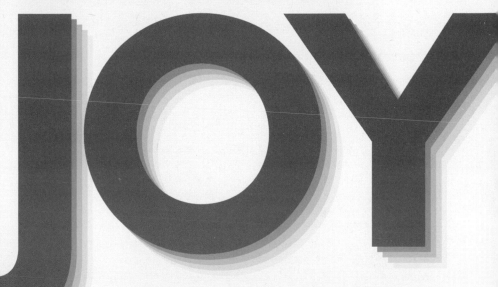

Trade Shame, Guilt, and Fear for Lasting Change,
a Lighter Spirit, and a More Fulfilling Life

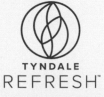

TYNDALE
REFRESH™

Think Well. Live Well. Be Well.

Visit Tyndale online at tyndale.com.

Visit the authors online at https://enjoycowellness.com.

Tyndale and Tyndale's quill logo are registered trademarks of Tyndale House Ministries. *Tyndale Refresh* and the Tyndale Refresh logo are trademarks of Tyndale House Ministries. Tyndale Refresh is a nonfiction imprint of Tyndale House Publishers, Carol Stream, Illinois.

Start from Joy: Trade Shame, Guilt, and Fear for Lasting Change, a Lighter Spirit, and a More Fulfilling Life

Edited by Stephanie Rische

Published in association with the literary agency of Legacy, LLC, 501 N. Orlando Avenue, Suite #313-348, Winter Park, FL 32789.

For information about special discounts for bulk purchases, please contact Tyndale House Publishers at csresponse@tyndale.com, or call 1-855-277-9400.

To protect the privacy of our clients, the names and details of our case examples have been changed. All names are fictional, and any resemblance between the composites and real people is coincidental.

Library of Congress Cataloging-in-Publication Data

A catalog record for this book is available from the Library of Congress.

ISBN 978-1-4964-6665-5

Printed in the United States of America

28	27	26	25	24	23	22
7	6	5	4	3	2	1

To our son, Jude.

You are the best teacher of joy.

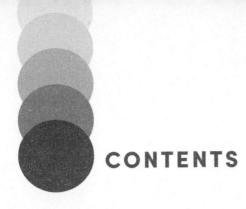

CONTENTS

INTRODUCTION What Does It Mean to Start from Joy? *1*

PART ONE The Start-from-Joy Life

CHAPTER 1 The Gifts of Joy *15*

CHAPTER 2 End the Motivation of Shame, Guilt, and Fear *31*

CHAPTER 3 Be Curious with Your Emotions *43*

CHAPTER 4 Interrupt Your Loops *63*

CHAPTER 5 Challenge False Scripts *81*

CHAPTER 6 Call Out the Judge *105*

CHAPTER 7 Find Your Joyful Purpose *119*

CHAPTER 8 Make It Fun *137*

PART TWO Empowered for Joy

CHAPTER 9 Enjoy Your Health *155*

CHAPTER 10 Enjoy Your Money *171*

CHAPTER 11 Enjoy Your Work *187*

CHAPTER 12 Enjoy Your Relationships *207*

CONCLUSION The Goal of Positive Change *227*

Acknowledgments *232*

Notes *235*

About the Authors *243*

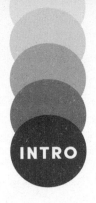

INTRO   WHAT DOES IT MEAN TO START FROM JOY?

How you start anything matters.

Starting your day at a frantic pace paves the way for greater stress, anxiety, and exhaustion as the day goes on. Starting a road trip with the wrong directions will likely lead to frustration and wasted hours of travel. Starting your workday with the steady drip of news and notifications from your phone will probably lead to less productivity and few results at the end of the day.

The same is true when it comes to our journey to positive change. As we embark on our quests to move our lives forward in meaningful, productive ways, it matters where and how we start. It can determine whether we get to where we want to go.

As professionals dedicated to helping individuals enjoy positive change, we've seen this truth lived out time after time. Moving our lives forward should be a fun and enjoyable experience. Yet people start their journeys from places that sabotage the good they want to accomplish. Instead of going to the gym for the fun of it, we treat it as a chore—a necessary evil in order to lose weight. Instead of starting new relationships with passion and excitement, our past baggage taints the thrill and poisons the hope of something new. Instead of crafting our own definition of parenting, we fear we'll be repeats of our parents who hurt us, which makes parenting even more difficult. In our work, we help people find a new starting point in their quest for positive change so they can reclaim the joy that leads to lasting, fulfilling results.

No example illustrates the power of starting points more clearly than this tale of two entrepreneurs.

The first entrepreneur was starting a business that should have been a raging success. It was in a booming industry, and he was addressing a clear felt need with his services. Yet he believed that to be a success, he had to keep the chip on his shoulder. He grew up watching big-time entrepreneurs point to a certain pain from their past as the launching pad for their endeavors. He, too, believed that he had to prove the world wrong. All this did was feed his shame of not being enough, his fear of messing up, and his guilt over not being more available for his family. This strategy worked . . . for a while. He was able to bulldoze his way into achieving some results. But the change didn't last. The desire to prove the world wrong turned into patterns of burnout, frustration, and hopelessness. Eventually, his business ended, crippled under the weight of shame, guilt, and fear.

The second entrepreneur had a different starting point. He didn't feel like he had anything to prove. In fact, his future felt full of hope, possibility, and wonder. His business was starting in an industry with various complications and regulations. On top of that, this was an entirely new industry for him. But this didn't deter him. With his energy and excitement, he inspired others to follow his vision, and he was able to build something that's still growing.

While the first entrepreneur started from a place of shame, guilt, and fear, believing his business would prove his worth and rescue him and his family from poverty, the second entrepreneur started from a place of joy, which led to lasting results. I (Neal) know their stories clearly because they're both mine. I am the entrepreneur who botched his first business, but I'm also the entrepreneur with a company that began the opposite way: from a place of joy.

THE SPARK FOR LASTING CHANGE

No matter who you are—whatever your relationship status or job title, whatever your financial situation or health condition, whatever your family of origin—we all have at least one area of life we want to change. We all have an area where we feel stuck.

Maybe you want to pay off your credit card debt, or maybe you want more energy throughout the day. Maybe you want to stop yelling at your kids, or maybe you want to stop dating jerks. Maybe you want to get into a regular workout routine, or maybe you want to stop your mind from going into overdrive every time something unexpected happens. We all have parts of our lives we want to change.

Unfortunately, breaking old patterns and pursuing change isn't something that comes naturally for most of us. We repeat familiar pathways, never seeing results, until any hope of change drifts away. Our credit card debt grows bigger. Our energy level wanes. Our kids continue to see the worst of us. Our dating prospects bottom out. Our workout routines turn into Netflix binges. And our minds spin in a cycle of anxiety.

Why is this so often the story for desired change? Why do we end up in a place of burnout, frustration, stress, and anxiety instead of the fulfillment of our dreams? Why does change seem so *hard*?

Many people would say it's an issue of willpower. Self-help gurus—the people who make fortunes from telling us what to do—might say, "You must not want it bad enough." But something about that doesn't ring true. You know more than anyone else how desperately you want to change.

Others would reduce positive change to a math problem. They might say you need to examine the components of your day to find the perfect formula for success. But you know it's not that simple. You've tried all the systems and methods for lasting change, and you're still here.

So if change isn't brought about by willpower or a magic bullet, what is it prompted by? Based on our years of professional experience and more than half a decade of study, we've landed on a simple conclusion: positive change is sparked by joy.

Not "Try harder." Not "Put your nose to the grindstone." Not "You should be ashamed of yourself." Not "Do it or else." Not "You should be past this by now." *Joy*.

Nothing is more motivating than our emotions, whether positive or negative. Emotions move us. Think about the biggest decisions you've made in your life—maybe it's going to a certain school or getting married or following a particular career path. Those decisions aren't just motivated by reason, right? They're also fueled by powerful feelings.

Yet we often ignore the role of emotions in building the life we want. While focusing on changing our thoughts and actions, we mistakenly lean on disempowering emotions like shame, guilt, and fear to create change. Most of the time we don't even realize we're doing it. But the white noise in our brains is constantly going something like this: *You're not good enough. You missed the mark again. You have to do better next time. That was stupid. What will happen if you don't get this right? You're so [insert shaming word here] for doing this again.*

But while negative emotions might prompt temporary change, after a while we'll slip back into our old patterns. Negative emotions are energy drainers that siphon the life out of sustainable change. The more we keep them around, the more we burn out and default to what we've done before.

There's only one emotion that will motivate lasting change and a more fulfilling life. This emotion is *joy*.

WHAT IS JOY?

Maybe when you hear the word *joy*, you imagine something cheesy and unconnected to real life, like a Disney movie or your gospel-singing aunt Sally. Or you might think joy is impossible and elusive in this season of your life. But the kind of joy we're talking about isn't dependent on your circumstances or your personality or your tendency to break into song at any given moment.

Instead, joy is a deep internal gladness inspired by hope, purpose, and delight. While happiness is based on our circumstances, joy is something we experience on an internal level. To reach for greater happiness, we have to change the hard parts of our lives. But joy is available at all times, regardless of whether we change our situation.

When we live from a place of joy, we don't *have to* change; we *get to* change.

This distinction makes all the difference when it comes to the hard parts of our lives. Instead of carrying the heavy weight of shame, guilt, and fear in the quest to change, we can live with joy regardless of whether we achieve the results we're hoping for. And it's precisely from this place that we can make changes that last.

WHICH COMES FIRST: CHANGE OR JOY?

This idea of starting from joy might sound simple, but there's one problem: many of us believe joy is the *result* of positive change, not the cause of it. We think that once we lose those pesky ten pounds, we'll be happy. Once we're out of debt, we'll be happy. Once we have a fulfilling job, we'll be happy. Once we're married, we'll be happy.

I (Neal) once bought into this mistaken idea. I believed that happiness was on the other side of painstaking change. If I put in the extra hours at work each day, then I'd be happy. If I shamed myself for not being a good husband, then I would change and be happier. If I was disciplined with my workouts, then I would find happiness. I thought that change came before joy—that I had to make change happen to finally enjoy life.

When we live

from a place of joy,

we don't *have* to change;

we *get* to change.

I know I'm not alone in this thinking. In a culture of self-improvement, we assume that the way to build an enjoyable life is to measure up, do more, try harder, run uphill, and white-knuckle our way through change. We've bought into the idea that change should be hard and painful, but that it's the only way to one day arrive at joy.

So we put ourselves to work.

We count calories and force ourselves to go to the gym, believing that thin equals happy.

We drag our feet to the office, believing we'll be happy once we get the promotion.

We deprive ourselves of entertainment, believing that we don't deserve to have fun until we've paid off that overwhelming debt.

We believe that joy is only possible on the other side of immense pain. We think that one day we'll have an enjoyable life, but only after putting ourselves through the work of difficult change. We've been sold the narrative that joy is a destination. If we stay the course and don't slip up, we'll "arrive."

This approach is sabotaging us. The reality is, we can't pursue positive change from a negative space.

Of course, it's true that we can hustle our way to results for a time. But as we crack the whip harder to achieve, we ignore the needs of our bodies. This is not sustainable, and eventually we will crumble under the weight. Negativity produces more negativity, and our efforts at change will eventually implode.

How we begin is how we end. If we force ourselves to change with feelings of shame, guilt, and fear, that's all we end up with. Starting from joy, on the other hand, puts empowering emotions at the center of positive change. This is the key to making change last: recognizing that joy is not the result of change but the cause of it.

Joy → Change

In his book *The Happiness Advantage*, positive psychologist and researcher Shawn Achor explains that success doesn't come before happiness. He says this "work hard for happiness" formula is backward. In reality, he says, it's the other way around.[1] It's only when we start from joy that we can experience lasting positive change and truly enjoy our lives.

THE PATH TO CHANGE

Starting from joy is not the default for most of us. We're used to motivating ourselves with emotions like shame ("Ugh, I'm so bad for eating that donut"), guilt ("I need to work off what I ate last night in the gym"), or fear ("I need to cut up my credit cards or I will never get out of debt").

We're used to stuffing our emotions at work so we can put up with the pain of going to a joyless job ("I'll be stuck in this dead-end job forever, but it's my duty to my family").

We're used to depriving ourselves of fun and delight in our relationships ("The last thing I want to do is go on a date after a long day at work").

We're used to going through the motions at church and feeling guilty for not praying or reading our Bibles more ("I feel like I'm not spending enough time with God").

We attempt to solve the hard parts of our lives with discipline, rigor, and extreme effort. We double down on a diet or a workout program, we restrict our money, we strive for hyper-productivity at work, we overlook daily moments of connection in pursuit of big dates and vacations, and we make our faith a series of to-dos.

But this mindset often backfires. Heavy restriction leads to bingeing. Doubling down on rules and regulations leads to injuries and exhaustion. Stuffing our emotions leads to eruptions. Sacrificing small, consistent moments of intimacy leaves us emotionally bankrupt. And guilt-based religion denies us a meaningful journey of faith. These aren't failures of not trying hard enough or not knowing enough; instead, they're the result of unhealthy emotional patterns. We don't arrive at the results we want because we're not feeling the right emotions from the beginning.

The negative emotions of shame, guilt, and fear sabotage the life we want. If we want to enjoy life, change needs to start from joy.

With a start-from-joy approach:

- Your reason to change isn't because you believe the worst about yourself or because you're trying to measure up. This is shame, and it will lead only to self-loathing.
- Your reason to change isn't because you did something "wrong." This is guilt, and while healthy guilt has its place, you will be dissatisfied in your journey if you remain stuck there.
- Your reason to change isn't because you're afraid of what will happen if you don't. This is fear, and while fear can lead to wise action, it will end up paralyzing you if it's calling the shots.

A start-from-joy approach isn't about "should" or "ought to" or "or else." Instead, it's the pathway for change that is fun, meaningful, and hopeful.

A FULLER LIFE AHEAD

When I (Neal) started doing this work myself, I thought, *I can't make change last, but I don't struggle with shame, guilt, or fear. Surely that's not the reason.*

But the truth is, these emotions are subtle, silent saboteurs. We often don't even recognize their role in our decisions and behaviors. We think that critical voice in our head is telling us the truth about ourselves. We assume guilt will lead us to do better next time, but in reality, guilt is not a place to stay. We don't realize we're motivated by fear, yet we're consumed by thoughts about what will happen if we don't change. Shame, guilt, and fear sneak in and slowly steer us into a negative, hopeless place.

When we start from joy, we choose a different motivation. It's not just a mindset shift; it's a *feeling* shift.

Starting from Shame/Guilt/Fear	Starting from Joy
I meticulously track my calories and exercises because I really need to shed a few pounds in order to feel good about myself.	I can learn to enjoy working out. It doesn't have to feel like a chore. I can celebrate progress and the mental and physical benefits beyond how I look.
I feel guilty because I know I should be reading my Bible more.	I can connect with God in a variety of different ways. And I can enjoy it!
"Savings September" just rolled into "Opt-Out October" and "No-Spend November." Guess I won't be getting together with my friends until the New Year.	It's possible to feel confident and empowered when it comes to money. I feel permission to save and to spend because I have a realistic plan in place.
I have entirely sworn off sugar. I throw away any sweets that come into the house because I'm afraid of what I would do with them.	I feel the freedom to eat a variety of foods without fear of losing control. I view food as something to be savored and enjoyed.
I need to put in extra hours at work or I'll never get the promotion I'm hoping for. Besides, I don't want to let my coworkers down. I have no work-life balance, but this is the only road to success.	I can trust that the work will get done while I honor my limits. Doing my job when I'm well rested and when I have healthy boundaries in place will lead to more positive outcomes, at work and at home.
My spouse and I are pitted "you versus me" on just about every subject. I feel like I'm alone in this marriage, and I'm afraid I will never get the love and respect I deserve.	I trust that my spouse and I can be on the same team rather than act as opponents. We can have difficult conversations to get on the same page, and our relationship will be better for it.

When we start from joy, lasting results follow. We know, because it's been true for the two of us, and it's been true for people we've worked with.

Like our client Nate, who conquered agoraphobia by challenging his fear-driven response.

Or Chelsea, who stopped speaking the worst about herself and found fun and enjoyment in going on dates.

Or Audre, who examined her relationship with exercise and made it a joyful experience instead of something to endure.

Or Violetta, who stopped overspending out of guilt and instead focused on creating meaningful experiences with her daughter.

Or Jordan, who found his dream job once he let go of his shame-inducing beliefs about the type of job he "should" have.

There's a fuller life ahead of you, one that's buzzing with joy. If you feel burned out and hopeless about your life ever changing, you don't have to stay stuck there. And if you don't feel stressed and frustrated but aren't experiencing the kind of transformation you'd like, there's a fuller life in store for you, too. No matter what you're wrestling with, joy is the secret to lasting positive change.

Carly and I are so passionate about this approach to change that we have poured our lives into helping other people experience it too. For over half a decade, we've studied psychology, therapy, neuroscience, and the Bible to develop a therapeutic approach to making lasting change—one that gives you practical shifts to combat disempowering emotions and help you embrace joy instead.

In this book, you'll learn the seven principles behind this approach and how you can apply them to different areas of your life, including health, money, work, and relationships.

- If you know the healthy choices you should make but struggle to execute them, this book is for you.
- If you start on the path to positive change only to burn out, this book is for you.
- If you repeat old patterns instead of breaking them, this book is for you.

- If you beat yourself up for not making the changes you want to make, this book is for you.
- If you're familiar with failed cycles of dieting, budgeting, and self-control, this book is for you.
- If you're exhausted from continually hustling, doing more, or trying harder, this book is for you.
- If you've read all the books and tried all the methods and you need an approach to change that works in the real world, this book is for you.
- And if you're wondering how your mental and emotional health intersects with your faith, this book is for you.

It's time to flip the script and try a lighter, more freeing approach to change. Instead of reaching for joy by putting yourself through intense change, put your joy first and lasting results will follow.

When you learn to start from joy, you'll end with joy. In doing so, you'll create an enjoyable and fulfilling life—the kind that ripples out into the world and brings heaven down to earth.

PART ONE

The Start-from-Joy Life

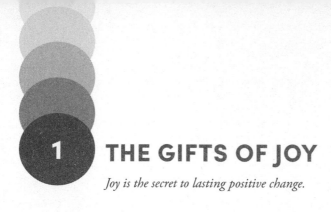

1 THE GIFTS OF JOY

Joy is the secret to lasting positive change.

"You should go to therapy."

Carly and I were at the tail end of an argument in our kitchen when she dropped this bombshell. We'd been in this argument before: I would feel pressure in my business and want to talk about it with Carly. She would feel helpless and stuck about how to advise me, and I would get mad at her for tuning out. Carly didn't know of a way to get past this issue besides asking for help.

You'd think being married to a therapist would make me more open to therapy. It didn't. I had no desire to sit in the office of a stranger and admit something was wrong.

But I also knew she was right. I was unhappy, frustrated, and stuck, and I didn't know why.

On the surface, I had everything that should have made me happy. I had a successful business, and I'd achieved my goals for the year. I'd tripled my income, and I had a steady flow of clients. I had a wife who was able to freely explore her passions and callings. I was able to provide for our family. I tried to tell myself those trophies were proof that I didn't need help. But after a few months of pretending nothing was wrong, I finally caved and scheduled an appointment.

As I sat in the waiting room to see a therapist named Myron, I stared at my feet, my phone, and the carpet, trying to prepare myself for what would take place behind that door. Did I mention I wasn't looking forward to therapy? As an entrepreneur, I was accustomed to meeting with business coaches. I looked forward to my meetings with them. They would pump their fists and shout, "We're going to crush our goals!" Those sessions were as thrilling as a rock concert.

Therapists, on the other hand, know how to kill the mood. I was sure I would hear, in the softest tone, "Get ready to do some *hard work*. It's going to be hard . . . so hard. But it'll be worth it." This didn't have me doing somersaults into the therapy room.

But Myron instantly shattered this misconception. When he opened the door in the waiting room to invite me back to his office, his smile caught me off guard. It was a wide, full-teeth smile—the kind a joyful, naive kid would offer. I'd been expecting an old man with narrow eyes that would examine my soul or something. Instead, Myron was full of life. My defenses fell.

I followed Myron through winding hallways and the *whirr* of white-noise machines until we came to his office.

As soon as I sat on the couch, I launched in. "I've achieved all my goals this year and built the business I wanted. So tell me—why am I not happy?"

Myron seemed unfazed by my attempts at impressing him. He proceeded to ask me questions about my childhood, my brothers, and my parents. He drilled down on where I'd learned certain beliefs and how they were playing out in my life.

After seeing him for several sessions, he pointed out the reality that was obvious to him—and was becoming obvious to me, too.

"It seems you've lost joy," Myron said one day.

I had no way of knowing in that moment what a journey those words would spark in me.

"WHAT'S WRONG WITH ME?"

Just down the road from Myron's office is another therapy office—mine (Carly's). As a therapist, I've met with countless people who have lost their joy—people who are spinning with anxiety, sinking in depression, and feeling more stuck than ever. I started my training by learning about cognitive behavioral therapy (CBT) and motivation-and-behavior change in addiction. I'd been trained to use motivational interviewing to combat these very issues. But something still felt missing in my understanding of positive change.

People would come to me and say, "Carly, no matter how much I change about my life, I feel like God doesn't love me. I don't love myself, and I'm just searching for the next thing to make me happy."

I knew what they meant. They believed something was barring them from greater joy in their life. But what was it? I put on my detective hat and began to explore what was behind this feeling.

I learned about more practices, including Emotionally Focused Therapy (EFT) and Eye Movement Desensitization and Reprocessing (EMDR). These practices helped me "refile" traumatic memories to where they belong so they have less emotional charge in the here and now. As I brought these modalities into the therapy room, I started to see that the barriers that were blocking people from joy were shame, guilt, and fear, and these emotions were deeply embedded in their personal stories.

I help clients change the question from "What's wrong with me?" to "What happened to me?" so they can heal the shame, guilt, and fear intertwined with their stories. It takes time and work, but people experience so much joy and freedom when they begin to loosen the chains of hurt and trauma that have held them down for so long.

I didn't realize it at the time, but this work would become the foundation of something Neal and I would build together.

THE FOUR GIFTS OF JOY

If you had told me (Neal) years ago that I would one day be the CEO of an emotional health-and-wellness company, I wouldn't have believed it. But here I am, years after Myron told me I'd lost joy, running a company that empowers people to find joy in their lives. At our company, Enjoyco, we believe positive change should be a fun, enjoyable experience from the start. We help our clients start from joy so they can create lasting positive change in their lives.

Back in Myron's office, his statement sparked curiosity in me. *Why joy?* I wondered. I began doing research, diving deep into the work of positive psychology, studying people like Martin Seligman, Mihaly Csikszentmihalyi, Barbara Fredrickson, and more, and also finding out what the Bible says about joy (God created it, after all).

At the dinner table, I would excitedly tell Carly what I'd learned about joy, and we would geek out together. She had a unique perspective, as she was seeing these principles come alive in the therapy room.

In those early days, we asked ourselves some probing questions:

- Why is joy the key to lasting change?
- Why does joy lead to a fulfilling life?
- Why is it important to cultivate joy at the onset of change?
- Why does change start with joy rather than some other mindset, such as peace?

We knew solving these questions was pivotal to unlocking positive change.

After years of asking ourselves these questions and seeing the principles play out in Carly's therapy room, we identified four gifts that

**Positive change
should be a fun,
enjoyable experience
from the start.**

are unique to joy. These gifts are what make joy the most empowering emotion in creating lasting change.

The four gifts are

- resilience,
- contentment,
- trust,
- and play.

Resilience

Resilience helps us withstand all the emotions of positive change.

We might think of positive change as being about our actions, but at its core it's really an emotional matter. That's because our actions are ultimately the by-product of how we feel. Most self-help gurus would advise us to put aside our emotions and fight our battle with mental toughness and fortitude. But this advice inevitably ends up being counterproductive. It creates an unhealthy relationship with our emotions, and having a flawed relationship with our emotions will sabotage our efforts to change faster than anything else.

Joy, on the other hand, helps us own the full range of our emotions. In doing so, we become more resilient when experiencing the emotions we don't want to face. It's the fear of "negative" emotions that causes us to sabotage ourselves. If we escape uncomfortable emotions that are essential for growth and change, we bar ourselves from the life we want.

The reality is that the road to positive change sometimes involves hard emotions. Change *is* uncomfortable—even when it's change we want. Joy acknowledges this reality and gives us the resilience to persevere instead of self-sabotage when the going gets tough.

In his book *The Voice of the Heart*, author and counselor Chip Dodd describes eight core emotions: hurt, loneliness, sadness, anger, fear, shame, guilt, and gladness.[1] He argues that when we feel these emotions in a healthy way, we can experience them as gifts. This means there's a good side to all our emotions.

- Hurt can lead to healing.
- Loneliness can lead to intimacy.
- Sadness can lead to acceptance.
- Anger can lead to passion.
- Fear can lead to wisdom.
- Shame can lead to humility.
- Guilt can lead to forgiveness.
- Gladness can lead to joy. (Hey, look! It's joy!)

Did you notice that all these emotions except gladness sound terrible at first? But Dodd argues that all of them are valuable because each one can lead to a positive outcome. There's a reason gladness and joy are at the bottom of this list, under the "negative" emotions. It's because true joy is possible only when we open ourselves up to feeling the other emotions.

You can't have the fullness of joy without risking the potential for pain.

Think about it this way: when you first learned to walk, you had no idea how it would turn out for you. You stood up on your wobbly two legs, put one foot in front of the other, and then . . . you fell flat on your face. Your parents might have rushed over, but you stood up again. You took another step and face-planted onto the carpet again. You kept repeating this until you experienced success. You learned to walk, but only after experiencing pain.

Carly and I recently became parents of a baby boy. Shortly after he was born, there were times when all I could do was watch him sleep. Other parents told me to "sleep when the baby sleeps," but I couldn't help but stare at my little one with immense love. I experienced so much joy partnering with Carly to bring this child into the world, but at the same time, I felt so much fear. I didn't want anything to happen to my son.

I wondered how this tiny human could render us so utterly vulnerable. We could have avoided this fear and vulnerability by not having a child, but we also would have missed out on the joy of experiencing this kind of love. Someone once told me that being a parent is like reaching the summit of the highest mountain, only to realize you're scared of heights. Now I know what they meant.

To rise to the heights of joy, we have to risk the possibility of falling.

Brené Brown calls joy the most vulnerable emotion. To experience joy, we have to open ourselves up to the potential of losing it.[2]

Something unexpected happens as we open ourselves to negative emotions: we grow more resilient to them. This resilience makes us stronger, so we persevere in creating lasting change.

Contentment

Contentment helps us detach from the results of our efforts.

When we're really hoping for something in our life to change, it might sound counterintuitive to want to be less invested in the outcome. But when the results become something we *need* to accomplish, the pressure stifles us and births hard emotions rather than empowering ones.

Donna is one of the most joyful people Neal and I know. But if you heard her story without meeting her, you would assume otherwise.

In 2020, when the COVID-19 pandemic was beginning to ravage the world, Donna was admitted to the hospital. Little was known about this disease at the time, but that didn't shake her. Instead, she had an unwavering peace about her. After several days in the hospital, the doctors advised her to go on a ventilator to give her more breathing capacity. She said no. "Save it for the other patients," she insisted. The nurses and doctors were baffled by her confidence and peace. Soon after, Donna made a miraculous recovery.

Donna's experience gave her newfound purpose. Since her recovery, she has walked with families who have lost loved ones to COVID-19. The same confidence and peace the doctors and nurses observed when she faced her own health crisis is now helping other families heal.

This internal peace, one of the gifts of joy, is none other than contentment. It's being okay when everything around us is not okay. Contentment isn't about forcing happiness or pasting a fake smile on our face in hard situations. It's drawing strength from a place of steadfast hope. While the world around us may break, our internal world is unshakable.

When we feel frazzled by our circumstances, the temptation is to try to change those circumstances. We think the path to being okay internally will come when we change our external reality. But contentment doesn't depend on what's happening in our lives. This is how Paul in the Bible was able to have joy while he was in prison. He wasn't trying to force his way to freedom. He didn't need to change his situation to find satisfaction. He had the kind of contentment that allowed him to rejoice even though his circumstances were far from ideal.[3]

If our joy isn't dependent on a change in our situation, we don't have to be held hostage by something outside our control. Contentment allows us to have a lightness of spirit and frees us from the pressure of trying so hard to control the outcome. And this in turn helps us create lasting change.

Have you ever felt that the harder you try, the harder it is to change? That's because the gap between where we are now and where we want to be gives birth to shame, guilt, and fear. This makes change feel more difficult, which then prompts us to try harder until we burn out. It's a vicious cycle.

On the flip side, have you ever felt like you were able to change parts of your life you weren't really trying to change? It almost feels unfair, doesn't it? The same principle applies. When we have less stock in getting results, we feel less pressure. And with less pressure, there's less shame, guilt, and fear.

If we can be okay and have peace no matter the results, we can set ourselves free from the pressure of trying so hard.

Trust

Trust helps us build the confidence and hope we need to make changes.

Whether we realize it or not, we all put our trust in something. When it comes to change, we are told to trust the guidance of self-improvement programs if we want to achieve results. We are fed promises like "Follow these ten steps for guaranteed results" or "Lose ten pounds with our workout regimen" or "Follow this simple three-step solution to financial freedom." These programs assure us that if we do exactly as they say, change is in our future. But Neal and I see this strategy backfire all the time, because this kind of change simply isn't sustainable.

My (Carly's) client Ariel is a good example. She only knew how to feed herself healthy foods if she was following a diet. She wasn't attuned enough to her body to know what to eat without external guidance. Her lack of trust in herself led her to yo-yo dieting and chasing program after program to achieve short-lived results.

Now, I'm not against self-improvement programs—I've been through plenty myself. But we have to realize that these programs end up corroding our ability to trust ourselves.

Joy, on the other hand, gives us the gift of being able to trust ourselves.

You can trust yourself to know what your body needs for fuel and care.

You can trust yourself to know what to do with your money.

You can trust yourself to know what you need in a relationship.

Yes, you might need to learn some skills or mindset shifts, but ultimately you know yourself and what you need better than any plan does. If we fear what would happen if we went off the program, then the program is not giving us true hope. We experience real hope for change when we believe we know what's best for us and how to take care of ourselves.

In her book *Emotional Agility*, Dr. Susan David says, "To make decisions that match up with the way you hope to live going forward, you have to be in touch with the things that matter to you so you can use them as signposts."[4] Here's the problem: what matters to us gets drowned out by the noise of what our culture, our family, and our friends say is important, cool, and right. We end up forfeiting trust in our bodies and our values.

This isn't to say that we should only trust ourselves. We can and should trust external guides and mentors, too—but only after we've filtered our decisions through our values. Without careful consideration, we will allow our sails to be blown in the direction of the strongest wind, which doesn't always lead us to the destination we intended.

God promises to give us wisdom directly. James 1:5 says, "If you need wisdom, ask our generous God, and he will give it to you" (NLT). That means we can trust him to lead us—through his Word, through his Spirit, and through wise mentors and friends. We don't have to outsource our decision-making to a program or to someone else's values.

What we've learned from our research is that happiness is based on circumstances, while joy stems from something internal. We don't find joy from listening to all the external sources telling us what should matter to us. Joy helps us trust what we know is true so we can build the life we hope for.

Play

Play helps us stick to positive change.

Research in neuroscience, psychology, and human behavior all indicate that we repeat behaviors we find pleasurable. God designed us this way to ensure our survival. If we didn't enjoy eating food, being in relationships, experiencing intimacy, and more, we would fail to thrive as the human race.

If we stick to the things we enjoy, it makes sense that joy must come before positive change. Any change we want to make in life won't last if joy isn't present.

The other day my (Neal's) friend James told me he bought a house that was in a higher price range than his original goal. In the past, such a decision would have been paralyzing for him. Because of past financial trauma, his feelings about money were tied up with a lot of fear. But this time, while he was taking the decision seriously, he was at peace about it.

When I asked him what was different this time, he said, "I finally felt safe to play with my money. I had been making wise moves to heal my emotional relationship with finances, and I knew this purchase wouldn't destroy us. So I decided to make a move that would pay dividends in our joy and happiness, even if it didn't make complete rational sense."

James was learning one of the keys to a start-from-joy approach. Play allows us to take risks and make investments in our own happiness. Change isn't about sitting in the heaviness of life and staying steeped in negativity. We need moments of play if we want to stick to positive change. If James hadn't taken any risks with his money, he would have remained stuck in fear. As he learns to enjoy his money, he'll continue to make positive, lasting changes in this area.

Joy naturally helps us stick to positive choices for our lives. When joy is missing from our efforts to change, it leads us to burnout. It's like swimming upstream or sailing a ship against the wind—we can do it for a while, but soon enough, we'll exhaust ourselves. When we add play to our quest for positive change, we create lasting results.

●　●　●

The four gifts of joy—resilience, contentment, trust, and play—help us stick to positive change for the long haul.

- Without the resilience of joy, we bend and ultimately break with the uncomfortable emotions surrounding change.
- Without the contentment of joy, we keep hustling and trying harder but never achieve internal satisfaction.
- Without the trust of joy, we jump from program to program without fostering the attunement that leads to lasting change.
- And without the play of joy, we never risk, grow, or enjoy the change we're seeking.

These gifts are what make joy the most empowering emotion for our positive-change journey. So how can we cultivate this joy, starting today, regardless of whether anything has changed in our lives? How can we begin to implement a start-from-joy approach?

A NEW APPROACH TO CHANGE

In our culture of self-improvement, we're constantly told to do more, learn more, try a five-step formula, or search for the new program that will help us achieve results. Yet all these "solutions" focus on what happens with our hands and heads, while ignoring matters of the heart, where we find the key to lasting change.

Years before Myron told me (Neal) that I had lost joy, I was a wide-eyed young marketer who was just starting my first business. One of my early marketing clients was a fascinating older gentleman named Robert. Robert was the director of the longest study of adult life and happiness at Harvard. He and his team tracked the lives of 724 men for more than 75 years. They also studied the sons and daughters of these men. In their study, they discovered what makes for a meaningful life. The answer was simple: good relationships keep us happier and healthier.

Robert shared these findings in a TEDx talk in Boston, and I was backstage eagerly listening as he revealed his findings to the world.

I was familiar with his study because I'd combed through his speech to work on his marketing. As I listened to him from the greenroom, each of his points hit my ears like beats in a pop song. When the talk ended, there was a roar of applause.

Robert's talk ended up becoming one of the most-viewed TED talks in the world. The large-scale interest in this topic revealed something obvious: people want to feel happy.

This simple revelation has profound implications for positive change. We pursue change to feel happiness and joy. Whatever we're trying to achieve—whether it's getting out of debt, deepening our relationships, or growing in our faith—we're pursuing the goal because we believe there's greater happiness on the other side. Yet happiness is an emotional matter. We can't ignore the heart if we want to achieve the desires of the heart.

Chip Dodd puts it this way: "We are people with heart pains and heart problems which require heart solutions. However, we attempt to solve heart problems with intellect, willpower, and morality, which are no more effective for solving heart problems than a shovel is for cutting a board."[5]

Maybe you feel desperate to change and frustrated that you haven't been able to break your patterns. Maybe you've tried everything, and nothing has worked. If so, it's time to try a different approach—one that leads with the heart. Instead of burying your emotions in the journey toward change, bring them to the center. Instead of putting yourself through more pain, try a lighter approach. Instead of forfeiting joy now for joy in the future, cultivate joy in the present, without the pressure to change anything.

The start-from-joy approach is built on seven principles. They are:

End the motivation of shame, guilt, and fear.
Be curious with your emotions.
Interrupt your loops.
Challenge false scripts.

Call out the Judge.

Find your Joyful Purpose.

Make it fun.

This is not a step-by-step program, nor is it a formula for guaranteed success. Rather, these are shifts to help you end the toxic influence of disempowering emotions on your journey toward change. This is a way to end the hustle and prioritize joy instead.

There's no specific order for these principles either—you can jump in anyplace that resonates with you during a specific season.

If you constantly invalidate your emotions on the journey to change, you can learn the valuable skill of being curious with them. If you have trouble stopping your self-sabotaging patterns and shame yourself for them, you can focus on interrupting these loops. And if you feel like change simply isn't fun, you can make it fun. These principles are interrelated, dancing with one another to help you achieve the change that connects with what you need right now.

In part 1 of this book, you'll learn about each of these principles and how to shift your feelings and thoughts in this direction. You don't have to try them all, though being open to all of them will give you the best chance for creating change. Even if you apply just one of these principles, you'll be on the way to building lasting change, creating a lighter spirit, and living a more fulfilling life.

In part 2, you'll discover how these principles work in some of the hardest areas to change. You'll find out how a start-from-joy perspective can help you stop the cycle of self-sabotage and achieve lasting results when it comes to health, money, work, and relationships.

If you've tried it all and still find yourself stuck, it's time to try something new. It's time to start from joy.

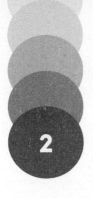

2 END THE MOTIVATION OF SHAME, GUILT, AND FEAR

*Instead of holding shame, guilt, and fear close,
end them for good.*

It was a chaotic day from the start. I (Carly) launched out of bed, realizing I was going to be late for work. I pulled on my boots and rushed out the door with a piece of toast hanging out of my mouth and coffee sloshing around in my cup. I could feel the tears welling up in my eyes as soon as I got in the car.

As I sped down the Boston highways, my anxiety was so palpable I could feel it under my skin. I trudged into my supervisor's office, catching a glimpse of myself in the windows. *Ugh, so disgusting,* my inner-critic voice said. The voice was so familiar that I thought nothing of it. When my stomach grumbled loud enough to shake the building, I gave it no mind.

I plopped down in a chair across from my supervisor, Amanda. She gave me one look, and I broke down crying.

I was in graduate school, working at an intensive addictions outpatient program and counseling agency. It was right after the Boston bombings, and I was seeing clients who were suffering from addiction and PTSD stemming from the trauma. On top of the stress I was feeling as I walked with people steeped in depression, suicidal ideation, and panic attacks, I was also trying to get good grades in graduate school and figure out life as a newlywed.

So I cried. A lot.

But if I was going to be crying, Amanda's office was a good place for it. Amanda was a small, quick woman with a fierce smile that said, simultaneously, "Everyone is welcome here" and "I could take you down if I needed to." She was the type of person who could both care for you and shoot straight with you.

I bawled my eyes out for a good three minutes before Amanda jumped out of her seat.

"I'll be right back," she said as she swiped a book off her shelf.

"Okay," I mumbled through my tears. I tossed tissue after tissue into her trash can, worrying that the pile would get so big it would topple over and leave a mess in her office. But before the tissues reached the top, Amanda charged back in.

"Your homework is to read this," she said, handing me a book with certain sections flagged.

I thumbed through the pages. It was a Brené Brown book with sections highlighting perfectionism and its relationship to shame.

"If you keep practicing therapy from a place of shame, you won't last," Amanda said.

This was the first time I learned that what I saw as my anxiety wasn't actually anxiety. It was something called shame. Brené Brown defines shame as "the intensely painful feeling or experience of believing that we are flawed and therefore unworthy of love and belonging."[1] That's exactly how I felt—like I wasn't enough. And this perception kept me performing, rushing, hustling, and doing everything possible to work my way into worthiness.

That moment marked the beginning of turning away from my

patterns of shame so I could start to see the joy in therapy instead. Without this shift in mindset, I wouldn't still be a therapist today.

THE APPEAL OF SHAME, GUILT, AND FEAR

When you believe joy is a destination you'll arrive at once you change yourself, your quest is likely to begin with shame, guilt, or fear. Your desire to change your life flows out of shame over not being enough, guilt over not doing enough, and fear of not having enough. Once you change everything that's wrong in your life, you think, *then* you'll be able to enjoy it.

But starting with shame doesn't lead to joy; it leads to more shame. That's how the pattern goes: shame begets more shame, fear begets more fear, and guilt begets more guilt. I've seen this pattern so many times now that I (Carly) can smell it in the air.

- I should read my Bible so I will be a good Christian. (shame)
- Because I ate this, I have to deprive myself of any foods I enjoy. (guilt)
- If I don't put in excessive hours at work, we will be poor. (fear)

We believe that being hard on ourselves will motivate us to pursue positive change. No doubt you've heard the phrase "No pain, no gain." We inflict pain on ourselves in our pursuit of change.

- When we skip the gym, we beat ourselves up with shame. We say, "I'm so lazy!"
- When we believe we've been "bad" in our eating, we wrack ourselves with guilt. We say, "I can't believe I ate that."
- When we have fears around money, we make self-sabotaging decisions, such as staying at a job we hate. We say, "I don't want to do this, but I have no choice."

We believe saying these things to ourselves will somehow whip us into shape and we'll start doing better. But as these emotions compound, they lead to a place of hopelessness, where we believe change is impossible.

Many of the clients I meet with are steeped in the "no pain, no gain" mentality. They believe that if they're too easy on themselves, they won't change. Yet staying in a place of pain motivated by shame, guilt, and fear is not productive. The truth is, *all pain equals no gain.* We can't shame, guilt, or scare our way into positive change.

When I was meeting with my client Ariel, whom I mentioned in chapter 1, she told me with vivid clarity about the moment she lost joy in her body. One day when Ariel was nearing puberty, she noticed that her gangly legs were growing stronger, her hair was beginning to shine, and she had some new curvature to her body. For the first time, she saw that she might look pretty. Ecstatic about the growth, Ariel ran to her mother. "Look, Mom! I'm pretty!" she said. "I'm growing!"

Her mom said, almost coldly, "You're not growing. You're just *fat.*"

In that moment, Ariel went from being in love with her growing body to feeling shattered. As she grew up, she struggled with eating disorders and a strained relationship with her body and exercise. As Ariel and I worked together, we discovered that she spoke to her body the way her mom had spoken to her body. She constantly called it fat, thinking this would inspire her to be better. She convinced herself that being too easy on herself would make change impossible. If she was happy with her body as it was, then she would never change. So she kept shame close to her chest. The constant belittling and self-hatred served a purpose—or so she thought.

The appeal of shame, guilt, and fear is that when it comes to getting results, they work—for the short term, at least. The problem is *how* this change occurs. When shame, guilt, and fear are calling the shots, we end up destroying our sense of self, wounding ourselves and others, and perpetuating patterns of anxiety and stress. Sure, this creates change, but it's not lasting, satisfying change. Even worse, we might achieve the result we wanted but not be able to enjoy it because of the means we employed to get there.

In a culture of productivity and self-improvement, we prioritize anything that gives us the desired results, even if it ultimately hurts us. We pay strict attention to the finish line, giving no mind to our feelings or the emotional patterns we're creating in the process.

Ariel kept her shame, guilt, and fear around because they helped her start the next diet. Every diet she committed to gave her fast results at first, but these results came at the cost of her self-esteem and happiness. She pushed through hunger cues, became militant about her food choices, and drained the joy from the room anytime she was eating with friends and family. She could only sustain this pace for so long before shame, guilt, and fear led her to self-sabotage.

The same goes for anything we try to change using shame, guilt, and fear. When we feel ashamed of our emotions, it leads us to bottle them up, only to have them erupt over small things. Guilting ourselves into reading the Bible and praying just fuels us with more guilt anytime we miss a day, and it moves our focus from intimacy with God to a series of to-dos. The intense fear of making the same mistakes our parents made keeps us from interacting with our children from a place of freedom and discovering the unique ways we parent. Shame begets more shame. Guilt begets more guilt. And fear begets more fear.

So why don't shame, guilt, and fear work for lasting change? There are two reasons.

The Brain Reason

There's a scientific reason why shame, guilt, and fear lend themselves to self-sabotage. Inside our skulls is a three-pound fold of tissue known as the brain.[2] God created this complex organ for a simple purpose: to help us survive. It does this by moving us toward pleasure. Think about it: if we didn't desire food, water, intimacy, and more, our species would be in danger. Many of the things that bring us pleasure are also essential for survival.

The brain also helps us survive by avoiding pain. If you saw a wild tiger, you would run, because the feeling of fear would prompt you to do so. You can thank your brain for that. This is called the law of approach and avoidance. We move toward the things that are good for us (pleasure) and away from things we perceive as bad (pain).[3]

The brain protects us from pain at any cost. And guess what? Shame, guilt, and fear are extremely painful emotions. Shame expert Joseph Burgo says that when we are ruled by shame, we build defenses to protect ourselves from experiencing it.[4] In an attempt to avoid shame, guilt, and fear, our brains often default to what brings fast relief, even if it harms us in the long run.

This was the case for my client Gina. Gina had a habit of falling for the "bad boy" who wouldn't be emotionally available for her. She feared rejection and being alone so much that her brain pushed her to keep going after these guys even though she knew rationally that it wouldn't work out in the end. She bought the false hope of "maybe it will be different this time," but she ended up self-sabotaging over and over again.

When shame, guilt, and fear enter the picture, the brain gets stressed. And when the brain gets stressed, it seeks relief. Neuroscientists have discovered that the stress of negative emotions puts us in a reward-seeking state.[5] We look for fast relief in anything that will help us *now*. The problem is, this wreaks havoc on our future selves.

When we use shame, guilt, and fear to motivate our results, we give more power to these emotions. And as these emotions increase, the brain's desire to escape them intensifies. We seek out faster solutions that end up reinforcing our inability to stick with change.

The self-help industry only reinforces this vicious cycle. According to most programs, if we just try harder or gain more knowledge, we'll be able to change. When we do try harder and learn all we can but still come up short, we believe there's only one possible solution: something must be wrong with *us*.

There are hundreds of thousands of self-help books that deliver actions and head knowledge alone to solve the issues we want to change. Of course, there's nothing wrong with action or information; it's just that they leave a piece missing from the puzzle.

For action and information to be effective, the rational part of our brain has to be working. There's a problem, though. The rational part of the brain—the neocortex, to be more specific—is the youngest, most recently developed part of the brain. And like a little brother who can never win against his older brothers, this rational part loses the battle against the emotional part of the brain whenever it gets stressed. That's why we jump to fast reliefs, only to beat ourselves up later for falling back into our old patterns.

Researchers Janet Polivy and C. Peter Herman made this discovery when looking at binge eating. They discovered that dieting often pre- cedes binge-eating behaviors. In their studies, they noticed that people on strict diets would inevitably "slip up" because, well, people were made to eat. They felt so guilty and ashamed of their lapse that they would binge eat. The researchers coined this as the "what-the-hell effect."[6]

Consider this example: A dieter eats a bite of cake and immediately feels guilty. Because guilt is painful, their brain wants to escape the feel- ing. So they escape by rushing toward the "reward" that made them feel bad in the first place. They say something like, "My diet is blown anyway. Might as well eat the entire cake." Then binge eating occurs. It's a classic example of how shame, guilt, and fear lead to self-sabotage.

The what-the-hell effect doesn't just affect dieters. When a person beats themselves up for missing a gym session, they may indulge in a Netflix binge instead. When a person shames themselves for spending more money than they planned, their whole budget may go out the window.

The reality is that being hard on yourself only makes change harder.

Being hard

on yourself

only makes

change harder.

The Biblical Reason

The science behind this cycle aligns directly with what the Bible says. In Matthew 25, we see the contrast between being motivated by joy and being motivated by shame, guilt, and fear. Jesus tells a story about a master who gives money to his three servants. The servant who is given the most invests the money and makes double in return. The servant who is given a little less invests it and also makes double in return. But the third servant does nothing with the money.[7]

It's clear that these first two servants start from a place of joy. The Bible describes them as going "at once" to invest the money and produce a return. Their excitement drives them to take a risk and pursue growth. What's even more interesting is that the servants could have lost the money they'd invested. But the result isn't what matters; it's the effort. They don't fear judgment from the master because they know the master and what he wants.

Sure enough, when the master returns, he celebrates the two who made a return. He invites them to "share in his joy." They start from joy and end up with more joy.

It's the third servant who doesn't know the master. When the master puts money into his hands, he's terrified. He feels like he has to guard the treasure, or else. He starts from fear and self-protection, and it leads him to play it safe and hide the money so he won't lose anything. When the master returns, this servant blames the master for his own failure to invest. Because of his misunderstanding of what the master wanted, he didn't end up with more joy like the other servants did. He ended up with more fear.

Too often we misunderstand what God wants from us. We chase after weight loss as if that's God's ultimate desire for us. We pursue greater wealth as if God put us on this earth solely to make money. We busy ourselves with trying to find a partner as if God's great commission is to find someone to spend our lives with. While these are positive aspirations, they're not what we were ultimately created for.

God entrusted us with blessings not so we can hoard them but so they can produce a return, for a bigger purpose. Understanding God's true heart and purpose for us leads us to more joy.

If we want to grow, we have to be like the first two servants, joyfully investing what we've been given. And when we start with joy in this way, we produce a return. We grow.

CAN SHAME, GUILT, AND FEAR EVER BE GOOD?

Maybe at this point you're thinking, *But isn't there a good side to shame, guilt, and fear? Aren't there times when those feelings are necessary?*

It's a valid point. If shame were all bad, how would we reconcile verses where Paul instructs a church to shame an unrepentant member?[8] If guilt were all bad, what would we do with the passages that talk about guilt leading people to seek God?[9] If fear were all bad, what would we make of the Bible's instruction to fear God?[10]

There's a distinction between a healthy version of these emotions and a toxic version. So what's that difference? Shame, guilt, and fear can be good *if* they produce the right fruit.[11]

The gift of healthy shame is humility—an acknowledgment of our limitations and a recognition of our need for Jesus. Toxic shame, however, leads to self-centeredness and even self-hatred.

Joseph Burgo says, "Productive shame focuses on discrete traits or behaviors rather than the entire person. Instead of making global statements about someone as completely worthless and irredeemable, productive shame leaves room for her to feel good about herself as a whole while also suggesting changes that might help her feel even better."[12] In other words, healthy shame affirms a person's value while leaving the door open for improvement. Toxic shame, on the other hand, shuts down hope. It reduces a person to their labels, placing their identity outside God's redemption. According to toxic shame, you are a sinner—with no hope, period. You *are* a cheater. You *are* a hypocrite. You *are* a failure. But that's not what the Bible says.

According to Scripture, everyone who believes in Jesus will not be put to shame.[13]

When we use shame to motivate positive change, we often think we are utilizing healthy shame that leads to humility. The healthy side of shame points us back to God and the hope we have in him. The toxic side of shame, however, points us back to ourselves. It says we're the saviors of our own lives. When we believe we're using healthy shame to motivate change, it's actually toxic, because we don't have the power to change hearts and minds the way God does. Toxic shame just reinforces the labels that shut down change.

The gift of guilt is forgiveness.[14] When we acknowledge that we have gone against God's best plan, the helpful action is to accept responsibility, take ownership, and receive forgiveness. If we never experienced healthy guilt, we would be sociopaths—never feeling remorse or acknowledging wrongdoing. While healthy guilt moves us into the productive action of forgiveness—both giving it and receiving it—toxic guilt burdens us into inaction.

With forgiveness comes transformation.[15] As teacher Adele Calhoun says, "Confession embraces Christ's gift of forgiveness and restoration while setting us on the path to renewal and change."[16] When we use toxic guilt to motivate positive change, we heap on the weight of self-condemnation rather than receiving the clean slate Jesus offers us.

The gift of fear is wisdom.[17] Without healthy fear, we would charge into battle without preparation. Toxic fear, on the other hand, leads to anxiety. When we're in a state of anxiety, we spiral in our thoughts, making too much of problems and draining ourselves of the energy to move forward in wisdom. While healthy fear leads us to acknowledge what's true, toxic fear keeps us stuck in lies and what-ifs.

When we motivate positive change with toxic fear, we get anxious about eating the "wrong" foods, fearful that one misstep will implode our entire weight-loss plan. We get anxious about our work, fearing that one mistake will mean the end of our jobs. We get anxious about our relationships, assuming false motives on other people's behalf.

There's a simple way to determine whether you have toxic or healthy shame, guilt, and fear, and that's to assess the fruit.

- Does your shame lead to self-hatred or to humility?
- Does your guilt lead to inaction or forgiveness?
- Does your fear lead to anxiety or wisdom?

* * *

Toxic shame, guilt, and fear aren't just a bad approach to change; they're a bad approach to living.

Amanda revealed to me (Carly) that I was practicing therapy from a place of shame. It showed up as perfectionism and doing too much of the emotional work for my clients. I felt I had to get results for my clients, because if they didn't change, what would that say about me and my worthiness? This pattern was leading me to burnout. Thankfully, I learned to recognize the shame fueling my patterns so I could interrupt this saboteur and make therapy fun again.

When we start from joy, we stop using shame, guilt, and fear as motivators. If you've been holding those emotions close to your chest, thinking they're producing a return for you, then it's time to drop them. Joy surpasses them every time.

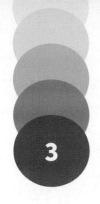

3 BE CURIOUS WITH YOUR EMOTIONS

Instead of feeling shame, guilt, and fear over your emotions, learn from them.

Rachel had a seemingly perfect life. She came from a good family with two present parents who showered her with love. Growing up, she had everything she could have wanted, and nothing particularly bad happened to her. She excelled at school and graduated with a deep pocket of friends and a streak of good grades that could get her into any college she wanted to attend. In college, she dove deeper into her relationship with God. Once she graduated, she quickly secured her dream job in Nashville's music industry. Everything seemed perfect, and everything about her looked perfect too.

But that's not why she was in my (Carly's) office.

"My mother always taught me to put my best foot forward," Rachel told me in our first session. "She taught me to trust God for everything, and I do. So why do I feel paralyzed by this awful anxiety?"

On the surface, you wouldn't be able to tell that Rachel struggled with anxiety. She was beautiful and put-together as she sat with straight posture on my therapy couch. But underneath she was being suffocated by anxiety. She dealt with a heavy case of "impostor syndrome"—feeling like she didn't belong at her high-end job. It was natural for her to feel anxiety in her position, but to her, this meant something was wrong with her. She wanted to get rid of the anxiety—fast.

Compounding Rachel's struggle was her reticence to explore her relationship to fear. If we want to grow, we have to accept that fear is part of any type of change. But Rachel didn't want to hear this.

"God hasn't given me a spirit of fear," she told me. "I shouldn't feel this way."

"Anxiety and fear are uncomfortable to feel," I said, leaning in. "But I'm curious, what do you think is underneath that anxiety?"

"It doesn't matter what's underneath," she immediately snapped. "Can you give me something to get rid of this?"

Rachel did her best to ignore or suppress her anxiety any time it popped up. When she couldn't do that, she blamed it on factors outside her control—everything from hormones to the weather. She was under the illusion that life should be *all* happy. The existence of a negative emotion meant something was wrong. She wanted to do everything she could to keep the negative emotions at bay, but this denial only made her more unhappy.

Studies show that people who suppress their emotions are less capable of repairing their negative moods. They experience fewer positive emotions and more negative emotions. Plus, they have lower life satisfaction and lower self-esteem.[1]

This was the case with Rachel. The more she downplayed her negative emotions, the more her self-esteem plummeted. She was unable to accept that as she grew older, took on more responsibility, and experienced negative emotions at work and in life, fear would be part of the picture. Life had been easy for her up to this point; she thought that if she just showed up with the right intentions and trusted God to provide, she would get the A. She'd impress the boss. She'd move up in her company.

When life got messy, and negative emotions entered the picture, Rachel assumed something was wrong with her. The trouble came not from the negative emotions but from her view of them.

TOXIC POSITIVITY

I (Carly) have met with several clients like Rachel who want nothing more than to jump out of pain and chase happiness. They are not alone in this—we are all uncomfortable with pain.

When something hurts, whether in our bodies or in our emotions, we want to move away from that pain. This isn't just a matter of culture or personality; humans are hardwired to keep chasing happiness. This is actually a gift, because fleeing pain can protect us from situations where danger is imminent. The trouble comes when we avoid all types of pain and don't deal with the underlying cause. If we avoid all painful emotions, we miss the opportunity to learn from them.

At their core, our emotions are neither positive nor negative. Dr. Susan David says that emotions "signal rewards and dangers. They point us in the direction of our hurt. They can also tell us which situations to engage with and which to avoid. They can be beacons, not barriers, helping us identify what we most care about and motivating us to make positive changes."[2]

Whether you consider yourself an emotional person or not, we are all emotional beings. If we spend a lifetime avoiding "bad" emotions and seeking only happy ones, our ability to experience positive change will be limited. The truth is simple: if we deny, suppress, or ignore one side of our emotions, we miss out on the change they can usher into our lives.

We are constantly pressured to force a false positive whenever we feel bad.

- Have you ever told yourself, *It's nothing*, and invalidated your negative emotions?
- Have you ever sat with someone who was hurting and tried to hurry them out of their emotions?
- Have you ever been scolded by someone to "just be grateful for what you have"?
- Have you ever spoken your heart to someone, only to hear the response, "It could be worse" or "At least you're not . . ."?
- Have you ever tried surrounding yourself with "good vibes" only?

These mindsets and behaviors are hallmarks of *toxic positivity*. Toxic positivity is the idea that only positive emotions are acceptable. This belief leads us to deny, suppress, invalidate, or rush out of negative emotions instead of sitting with them long enough to find healing. In a *Washington Post* article, psychologist Natalie Dattilo is quoted as saying that toxic positivity "results from our tendency to undervalue negative emotional experiences and overvalue positive ones."[3]

While this way of thinking might feel like a relief in the moment, it ends up doing damage in the long run. By avoiding all pain and negativity, we never actually confront the pain, and in doing so, we make it worse. It's like trying to submerge a fully inflated balloon underwater—it always finds a way to pop back up.

When we talk about a start-from-joy approach, it's important to clarify up front that this isn't about slapping on a happy face, forcing false positivity, or ignoring reality. You're not going to find any woo-woo positivity or "fake it till you make it" mindsets here.

We want to be very clear: a start-from-joy approach is *not* toxic positivity. It's not about running from hard emotions. It's not about being happy no matter what, and it's certainly not about suppressing or ignoring our negative experiences. If we shame, guilt, or scare ourselves out of hard emotions, our joy is the cost.

What Joy Is Not

The mistake we make about joy is believing it means rejecting our negative emotions and replacing them with fake positivity—the kind that denies reality. This interpretation is rampant throughout our culture, but it finds a unique home in the Christian community. We mistakenly assume that when the Bible talks about being joyful in all circumstances,[4] it means we're not supposed to experience negative emotions or allow ourselves to sit with them. We might feel pressure to tell ourselves and others, "God has a plan" or "God doesn't give us anything we can't handle." In reality, however, the Bible is full of examples of faithful people who lamented and who were honest before God with their full range of feelings.[5] If Christian joy were more like toxic positivity, we would see Jesus shy away from these emotions. Instead, the joy of Jesus always moves toward people and their pain, not away from it.

The Bible states that joy comes *after* feeling the fullness of our negative emotions. Take John 16, for example: Jesus tells his disciples they will weep and lament, but their sorrow will turn to joy.[6] He doesn't say they should ignore their sadness or move on as quickly as possible. He says they will feel the fullness of their negative emotions and joy will be on the other side.

One of the greatest obstacles to experiencing joy is our inability to sit with hard emotions. But when we accept that God himself sits with us in our pain,[7] we can give ourselves (and other people) permission to feel our feelings and pursue the path to true joy.

The Cost of Toxic Positivity

Leading neuroscientist Antonio Damasio was perplexed. His patient Elliot was carrying on a normal conversation with him. He was charming and pleasant during their interaction, and Damasio saw no red flags signaling that anything was wrong. Yet he was certain: something *had* to be off.

While Elliot carried himself well, his personal life was a mess. His first and second marriages had ended in divorce. He'd lost his job. The new business he started went bankrupt. He couldn't finish any projects. By the time Damasio found him, he was living with a family member after being denied disability assistance.

Elliot hadn't always been like this. In fact, he was once a model citizen. He had been revered at his job. He and his wife had a close, intimate marriage. And his family loved the man he'd been.

So what happened?

One day Elliot started to get headaches. Doctors discovered a tumor that was damaging the frontal lobe of his brain. He opted to have it removed, thinking that would mark the end of his troubles. Unfortunately, this was when many of his problems began. Following the surgery, Elliot became a different person.

As Damasio dug in, he found that Elliot struggled with decision-making. Though his intelligence, logic, and skills were still intact, he had no idea how to start and finish projects, execute plans, or make basic decisions. Damasio was struggling to connect the dots in his observations until he had a realization: he was studying the wrong thing.

Elliot's intelligence was still there. What was missing was his *emotional capacity*. Though he had his intellect and reasoning abilities, the absence of emotions made it nearly impossible for him to bring about any positive change. Logic alone, it turns out, ruined his life.[8]

Too often we fear our negative emotions, so we invite only our happy feelings into our pursuit of change. When we self-sabotage, we blame it on emotions and try to double down with willpower, self-discipline, and mental toughness. We don't realize that the reason we perceive emotions as unfamiliar threats is that we haven't dealt with them head-on.

- When we don't identify shame, it leads us to destructive behaviors.

- When we don't recognize guilt, it leads us to continually beat ourselves up.
- When we don't name fear, it leads us to hustle for control.

This is the cost of toxic positivity. If we never sit with hard emotions, we can never learn from them. And if we can't learn from them, we forfeit the resilience that comes with joy.

EMOTIONS AS SUPERPOWERS

Our emotions can be a tool for helping us learn and grow. The secret is to get curious about them. Rather than immediately jumping out of uncomfortable feelings, we can notice them, regulate them, and see what they're trying to show us. This skill will turn our emotions from a stumbling block into our greatest strength on the road to change.

Here's how to build this crucial skill in your life:

Name Your Emotions

"Where do you feel it in your body?"

That's what my (Carly's) first therapist asked me.

When I went to therapy in college, I was a blubbering mess. As I made my way through my therapist's box of tissues, I had no idea how to handle my emotions. I felt flooded, embarrassed, and relieved all at the same time.

I went to see her because I didn't know what to do about a boy I was dating. I had a feeling that maybe I should dump him, but as a young college student without much perspective, I felt like such a decision would make or break me. In my first session with my therapist, I let the emotions explode.

"What?" I asked through my tears.

"Where do you feel the emotion in your body?" she asked again.

At the time, I didn't understand what she was talking about. But looking back, I know exactly what she was leading me to.

Emotions are felt in our bodies. By identifying where we sense them, we can gain greater emotional awareness. It was clear that I had no positive relationship with my emotions. If I had, maybe I wouldn't have exploded like a shaken-up Coke bottle.

I started to compose myself. "Here," I said, putting the palms of my hands around my neck.

In the years since, I have learned to take note of my feelings and listen to what they're telling me. I know now that when I feel shame, it comes out in my neck, as if my voice has been stripped away. It's a signpost for me to pay attention, an external marker for what's happening on the inside. Now when I experience shame, I know how to recognize it, how to identify what the trigger is, and how to best respond in the moment.

We live in a society that tells us our feelings can't be trusted. We spend a lifetime shutting them down and shaming ourselves for them, not realizing that they have the capacity to empower us. When emotions are fully felt, realized, and processed, they can help us reclaim our sense of agency. When we are in a perplexing situation, our bodies give us a signal about what to do next. When we shut down this relationship to emotions, we are forced to react to them instead of lean into their wisdom. For example, if our bodies send us the signal of anger, we can know that a boundary has been crossed, and we can take wise steps to reclaim that boundary. Or if our bodies send us the signal of sadness and grief, we can pay attention to it and slow down. This allows us to read and respond to our bodies' signals instead of burying them and pursuing happiness at any cost.

Neuroscientist and researcher Lisa Feldman Barrett coined the term *emotional granularity*, the ability to accurately read and identify our emotional experience. People with low emotional granularity might label emotions like sadness and anxiety in broad terms, such as "I feel bad." People with high emotional granularity are able to identify with great specificity emotions like joy, sadness, anger, and shame.[9]

Emotional granularity helps us regulate our emotions because by accurately naming them, we can gain more power over them. One study found that people with higher emotional granularity are less likely to engage in self-sabotaging behaviors such as binge drinking and behaving aggressively when they experience emotional distress.[10] In other words, being specific with our emotions can save us from engaging in our protection responses.

When I ask my clients what they're feeling and they respond with a specific emotion, I follow up with another question: "And what else?"

My clients typically shoot me a questioning look at first, but after considering it, they are able to identify another deeper emotion.

We often feel one emotion on the surface, but that's not the emotion that's fueling our self-sabotage. What might feel like anger is actually fear underneath. What might feel like anxiety is actually unresolved sadness.

I once worked with a couple that had a recurring problem: the husband kept leaving their newly mobile baby alone in a room with their scared dog. The wife was furious at the husband for doing this, so she laid into him. He got defensive and lashed out in response. On the surface, the emotion both of them felt was anger.

When I asked them, "And what else?" they sifted through the noise and found the real painful emotion underneath.

"Shame," the husband answered.

"Fear," the wife answered.

The husband felt shame because he wanted to be a good father, and this stressor conflicted with his desired identity. The wife felt fear because she was concerned about her child's safety. On the surface, they both were experiencing anger, but their responses were being fueled by fear and shame.

Before you settle on an emotion, ask yourself: *And what else?* This powerful question can help you mine whether there's another emotion under the surface.

LIST OF FEELINGS

Nearly fifty years ago, psychologist Paul Ekman identified six emotions he said are shared by people in every culture. The list below starts with those basic emotions and then provides many more gradations. Though it is certainly not complete (and some feelings may cross categories), referring to this list may help you identify your feeling. Why is that important? Research shows that naming your emotion may calm your limbic system and support the integration of your brain.[5]

Happy	Sad	Angry	Fearful	Surprised	Disgusted
Amused	Blue	Agitated	Afraid	Astonished	Cynical
Carefree	Burdened	Aggravated	Alarmed	Confused	Disillusioned
Cheerful	Depressed	Bitter	Antsy	Curious	Disturbed
Excited	Despondent	Brooding	Anxious	Delighted	Embarassed
Exhilarated	Disappointed	Cranky	Brooding	Enchanted	Exasperated
Giddy	Discouraged	Cross	Cautious	Horrified	Fed Up
Grateful	Drained	Defensive	Despairing	Incredulous	Humiliated
Joyful	Gloomy	Frustrated	Frightened	Impressed	Jaded
Loved	Grief-stricken	Furious	Helpless	Inquisitive	Jealous
Merry	Hopeless	Hostile	Hesitant	Intrigued	Offended
Optimistic	Lonely	Impatient	Insecure	Mystified	Outraged
Relaxed	Melancholic	Rebellious	Nervous	Puzzled	Repulsed
Satisfied	Pensive	Resentful	Rattled	Shocked	Revolted
Thrilled	Remorseful	Scorned	Stressed	Skeptical	Scandalized
Tranquil	Troubled	Testy	Tense	Startled	Sickened
Upbeat	Weary	Upset	Worried	Wary	Smug

Regulate Your Emotions

The great benefit of accurately assessing emotions is that it helps us identify *less* with our emotions. When we feel a certain way, we say things like, "I'm sad" or "I'm mad." The reality is, we aren't sad; we're *feeling* sad. We aren't anxious; we're *feeling* anxious. We aren't angry; we're *feeling* angry.

The reason we feel flooded by our emotions is that we overidentify with them.[11] This overidentification makes it harder to regulate ourselves. We get swept away in our emotional experience and find it difficult to recover.

The goal of naming an emotion is to put a space between us and the emotion. Too often we believe we are our emotions. That's why we're afraid to give difficult emotions space. When we hold these emotions close to our chest, they become all-consuming, and all we can do is blindly follow their demands. But when we accurately label a feeling, we're able to add distance between who we are and the way we feel.

This distance is pivotal for positive change. For one thing, it allows us to identify what the emotion is tempting us to do. For example, whenever I (Neal) feel shame, I might say, "My shame is tempting me to overidentify with my successes and puff up my ego right now." Or I might say, "My fear is tempting me to procrastinate on this work." When I can articulate what is happening, I am one step closer to having the power to change it.

This distance from our emotions also helps us realize how fluid they are. Emotions come and go. We might feel a wave of shame and then see it wash away just as quickly as it came. If we can recognize a particular feeling, we'll be better equipped to ride it out.

After neuroanatomist Dr. Jill Bolte Taylor suffered a massive stroke, she began learning about her brain and recording her insights. She discovered that when we encounter a stressor in our environment, there's a ninety-second chemical reaction that happens in our bodies—our emotional response. Anything beyond that minute and a half is a choice to remain in that emotional loop. Dr. Taylor notes that if we encounter a stressor, we should wait for ninety seconds before responding. We can experience the initial response in our bodies and then watch it pass by. She calls it the ninety-second rule.[12] This isn't to say that every emotion you feel should only last for ninety seconds. Grief and trauma can sit in our bodies for a long time. Rather, the initial wave of a hard emotion comes and goes in ninety seconds.

The reason we stay on alert after ninety seconds is because our negative thoughts restimulate the process. The moment we add judgment to our thoughts (*I can't believe this is happening* or *I shouldn't be feeling this way*), more stress is pumped into our bodies. This loop gets repeated and demands increasingly unhealthy coping mechanisms to escape. We call this a Negativity Loop (more on this in the next chapter).

As we become mindful of what's happening inside our bodies, we can resist self-critical, judgmental thoughts and practice kindness toward ourselves. The next time you experience something negative, imagine your emotions as a child and yourself as a loving parent. Recognize the emotion, name it, validate it, and then watch it wash away. Then you'll be able to take a deep breath and get back to business.

For example, if I were suddenly triggered by someone telling me I did a bad job on a project, I might take a deep breath and say this in my mind: *It's okay. I'm feeling shame right now. My shame is tempting me to get defensive and fight back. But this is just a feeling I have right now. I'm going to watch this emotion wash away.*

Mine Your Emotions

Once you're in a place where you feel safe with your emotions, ask yourself, *Why is this emotion here? What value is this emotion pointing me to?*

Emotions can be signposts for what we value. As we mindfully explore our emotions, we begin to learn the values buried underneath.

If you felt angry when your friend criticized your work, there's a reason you got angry. It's not just because your friend was being a jerk. You might value putting out exceptional work, and your friend's criticism triggered you because it made you feel like you weren't living up to this value.

Uncovering our values helps us decipher the life we want to live. Instead of blindly reacting to situations, we can be proactive in creating a life we enjoy—a life that's in alignment with our values. In order to do this, we need to pay attention to what our emotions are trying to teach us.

Our emotions can be our teachers instead of monsters we try to escape. The key is to ask ourselves what the emotions say about us and what we value, once we've regulated them.

Let Your Pain Matter

It didn't take Myron long to see what was holding me (Neal) back from joy. From a young age, I'd had a pattern of emotional suppression. In my house growing up, it wasn't safe to feel our emotions. We were taught (by example, if not through words) that emotions lead to angry outbursts, fists, broken furniture, and police showing up at our door. Emotions were the source of great pain and distress.

After one such episode, when I was just ten years old, a family member came to help pick up the wreckage. I was quietly sobbing in the corner. This family member knelt down, wiped away my sniffles and tears, and said, "You know, the next time this happens, you shouldn't cry. Anytime you cry, you hurt your family more than they're already being hurt. You don't want to hurt them more, do you? Be brave."

Thus began decades of stuffing my emotions. The only emotions that felt safe to me were the happy ones.

Myron picked up on this after my response to several of his questions. "Doesn't that make you angry?"

"Not at all," I would reply stoically.

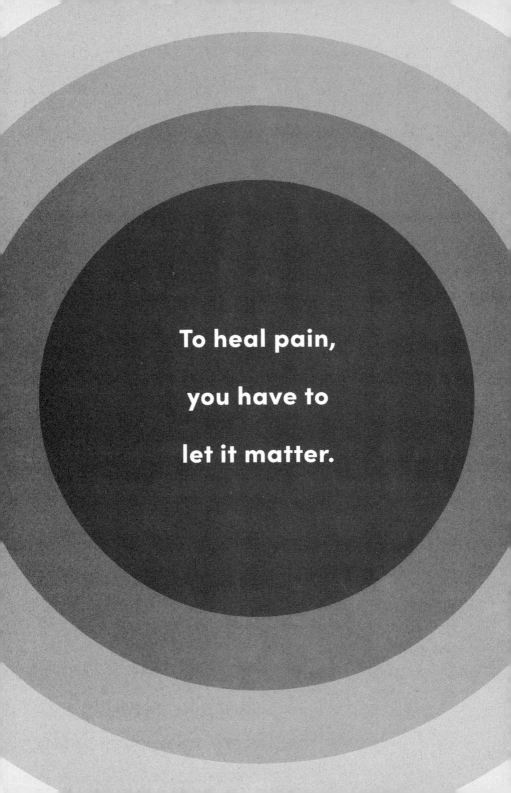

To heal pain,

you have to

let it matter.

Another time he said, "That sounds like it hurts."

"I guess."

And again: "If I were you, I would feel a lot of sadness and disappointment about that."

"Eh, I got over it."

My heart made a habit of invalidating my pain and siphoning the emotion out of it. This created a lifestyle of reacting to pain instead of addressing it.

Through my work with Myron, I learned a crucial truth: to heal pain, you have to let it matter.

Many of us spend a lifetime gaslighting our pain and pretending it's no big deal. We convince ourselves that we shouldn't feel anything other than happy and grateful. In this emotional suppression, we rush to self-sabotaging reliefs to feel better in the short term. As we do, we drift further and further from positive change.

In an attempt to make other people feel better, we may inadvertently minimize their pain too. Have you ever caught yourself saying something like this?

- "That's not the way you should think about that."
- "At least you're not . . ."
- "That's nothing compared to what I went through last week."
- "On the bright side . . ."

The healthy alternative is emotional validation—communicating that hard emotions are part of the human experience and that they make sense in the context of a particular story or set of circumstances. Studies show that acceptance helps validate our emotions and shows us we are valued as we are.[13] Validation helps us better regulate our emotions by lessening their intensity. If we feel heard and seen in our hard emotions, we feel safe, and thus move out of our distress faster.[14]

Imagine if Jesus had told those he met who were in pain, "Well, that doesn't compare to what I'm about to do for all of humanity." He didn't, of course. Instead, he acknowledged their hurt and touched them and empathized with them and wept with them. In other words, he validated the full spectrum of human emotions.

In the ultimate form of connection, Jesus came down from heaven in human form and experienced pain with us. He made space for the hurts of humanity. And it was in the context of this emotion-first approach that he ushered in massive transformation.

Sometimes we aren't able to offer ourselves the emotional validation we need. You might have grown up in a culture that was antagonistic to emotions or a culture that was prone to toxic positivity. Maybe to make others happy, you had to be happy yourself, which created a habit of pretending hard emotions weren't real. If this is the case for you, you can start by letting someone else validate your emotions for you.

I (Carly) often find that my clients struggle with validating their own emotions unless they have safe people in their lives who show them how. Emotionally safe people can help us accept our hurts, know that we're not alone in our pain, and realize that our pain matters.

Safe people—those who have earned the right to hear our stories and enter the deep places of our lives—give us emotional security. In this place of safety, joy can flourish. If we don't feel safe to experience our emotions, we'll never venture into uncomfortable territory to carve out new paths for ourselves.

Imagine being tuned in to a radio channel. It has crystal-clear reception, so you know exactly what's being transmitted from the other side. This is how emotional attunement works. It's the ability to understand and be present with someone else's emotions.

Here's what emotional attunement *doesn't* look like in your relationships:

- The person who tries to one-up your struggle: "That doesn't compare to what I went through last week!"
- The person who feels uncomfortable with your discomfort. They want you to be happy so much that they crumble when you're not.
- The person who won't let you feel your emotions. When you come to them with your pain, you end up having to comfort them instead.
- The person who invalidates what you're going through. "It wasn't that big of a deal. I'm sure you misinterpreted the experience."
- The person who tells you to toughen up and white-knuckle your way through the pain.
- The person who defaults to trite one-liners whenever they feel uncomfortable.
- The person who says, "I'll pray for you," and then gives you advice instead of praying.
- The person who only offers sympathy and never empathy. They say, "I feel sorry for you" rather than, "I feel with you."
- The person who tries to correct your thinking before connecting with your emotions.

A safe person, on the other hand, shows they are listening, responds in an appropriate way, reflects what you're feeling, and communicates that your pain makes sense. Here are the people to look for:

- The person who says, "That sounds difficult."
- The person who says, "It makes complete sense why you feel this way. What you're going through is hard."
- The person who says, "You're not alone in this."
- The person who says, "I'm with you."
- The person who says, "I can see why you feel this way."

- The person who says, "Mm-hmm" and "yes" to show they're tracking with what you're saying.

If you don't currently have a relationship with a safe person, consider seeking out a therapist or reaching out to a leader in your church. It's crucial not to let our emotions get brushed under the rug so we can move forward in our quest for change.

FROM NUMBING TO PURPOSEFUL PURSUIT

At the beginning of the COVID-19 pandemic, Carly and I were restless. The situation we'd thought would take two weeks to resolve was dragging on, making the future feel ominous and bleak. Around the same time, the lease on our house was ending. We weren't ready to buy a house yet but were itching for something new.

On a random day in April, we signed a lease on another house thirty minutes away. Though it was significantly smaller than the house we were living in, it had three bedrooms, which meant we could have a nursery—something that was important to us, as we were hoping to start a family. It was also within walking distance of both Carly's office and my office. It seemed perfect.

The night after we got the keys, I felt a restlessness in my spirit. That night a storm moved in and cut off our power for several hours. In the darkness and silence, I had the space to sit with my feelings, which was the very thing I'd been avoiding. I realized that moving didn't make sense for us at this point. We would be moving away from our community to a busy area, for offices we weren't even sure would stay open.

Suddenly it hit me: I wasn't starting from joy in this decision. Instead, I was starting from fear. I was feeling burned out in my job while also holding the uncertainty of the season. This combination of fear, anxiety, and exhaustion had led me to reach for something I could control, even if it wasn't the best decision.

The next day we were able to get out of our lease. Sure enough, both of our offices closed within the week. We were grateful to weather out the worst of the lockdown period in a familiar place, and then we had the flexibility to buy a house in an area that better suited our family the following year.

We often try to change our circumstances in an attempt to numb ourselves to the deeper pain in our lives.

Does work feel like a grind? Maybe it's time to switch careers.

Does parenting feel like an uphill battle? Maybe a bigger house will help your family spread out and get along.

Does your marriage feel like it's dragging? Maybe it's time to start a new diet so your spouse will notice.

When we feel the heaviness of life or when we're facing uncertainty, the temptation is to look for the next thing to make us happy. Even when the things we're pursuing are good, we may be pursuing them for the wrong reason.

There was nothing bad about wanting a three-bedroom house to fit our family. But this pursuit was tainted by the wrong motive. We were running away from what felt hard instead of pursuing positive change with intention and purpose.

When we heal our relationship with our emotions, we stop looking for quick fixes. We no longer need to seek control, numb our pain, or find the next bigger thing to make us happy.

If we're willing to learn from them, our hard emotions can help us turn inward, sift through the noise, and reattach ourselves to our deeper purpose.

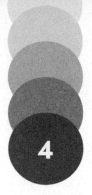

4 INTERRUPT YOUR LOOPS

Instead of shaming an unwanted behavior, interrupt your patterns.

Nate was a typical high school teenager in almost every way. He was on the shy side, approaching his seventeenth birthday. He would only open up if you garnered his trust. Then he would tell you all about his love for music. Living in Nashville, he soaked up every ounce of the music culture buzzing through the city. He spent all his free time playing around with music production, audio engineering, and songwriting. But there was one thing that set him apart from other teenagers.

He hadn't left his house in months.

It started his junior year of high school. For years Nate had struggled with the fear of judgment from his friends, teachers, and even strangers. This concern was manageable at first—he shrugged it off and reminded himself, *They're probably too busy worrying about themselves to care about me.*

Then Nate had a falling-out with his friends, which further spurred his anxiety. The anxious feelings followed him like a persistent ghost.

One morning, everything just felt off. He could no longer shrug off his anxiety. It didn't help that he hadn't been able to sleep the night before and had been awake until 3 a.m.

In class that day, his worry reached an all-time high. It started as a small pit deep in his stomach. His thoughts swirled with a constant undercurrent of anxiety. Then all at once, panic grabbed at his chest. His neck and shoulders shook, his heart pounded, and his eyes darted around, looking for an escape.

Thoughts zipped through his mind, rapid-fire. *What's happening? Is everybody looking at me? What are they thinking? Am I going to pass out? I think I'm going crazy. They're definitely looking at me. What if I fall and cause a big scene? What if they call an ambulance? What if I'm dying?*

He ran out of the room, collapsed on the floor, and had a panic attack in the hallway.

That was the last day he went to high school.

Nate's fear of having a panic attack in a place where he couldn't escape, physically or emotionally, is a symptom of what the therapy world calls *agoraphobia*. From that moment, he refused to leave his house. In fact, he never left his room. He was so afraid he would have a panic attack in public that he chose self-confinement, as if his room were the safest prison in the world.

Naturally, his parents were distraught. They tried to force him out, but this only triggered more panic attacks. So Nate stayed in his room, with depression weighing on him like a ten-ton elephant.

After his primary care physician suggested a thirty-day inpatient stay at a treatment center, Nate knew it was his time to take action. His parents found me (Carly) through a friend and set up an appointment.

It was a struggle to get Nate to come into the office. Most weeks he would give the same reason for canceling: he was too tired. He had so much anxiety over having another panic attack that he'd bail at the last minute. When he sent the cancellation text, relief would wash over his body, and he'd collapse in bed and sleep.

Over time, this became a pattern. We couldn't address his agoraphobia if he never came to see me, so I did some investigating to determine what was causing his tiredness.

After asking Nate some questions, I discovered he would stay up late watching YouTube videos, listening to new music, and playing around with music production until he fell asleep around four o'clock the mornings of our sessions. Nate was getting in his own way.

This is how self-sabotage works. Nate was too tired to fight off his anxiety, and then he was trying to solve the problem by staying up late (thus making him tired). It was a repeating loop. If he was ever going to change, this pattern had to be broken.

The same applies to all of us. If we want to stop defaulting to sabotaging actions in our pursuit of positive change, we need to understand our negative patterns and then acquire the tools to help us interrupt them.

THE NEGATIVITY LOOP

I can't believe I blew my budget again. I am such an idiot!

I said yes to going on a date with him again. Why do I keep going back?

This conflict is too much for me to handle. I don't want her to blow up at me, so I'll just ignore her.

We're used to shaming, guilting, and scaring ourselves whenever we take actions that contradict our goals. Yet this only disempowers us, sabotaging our efforts at change and making us feel hopeless. We grow apathetic and make jokes at our own expense, all the while repeating these negative patterns. If you want to see an example of this, go on Facebook or Twitter a week after people set New Year's resolutions. Studies show that most people who set resolutions give them up by February 1.[1]

In a survey by the American Psychological Association, people listed lack of willpower as the number one reason they couldn't stick to positive lifestyle changes.[2] But in reality, the problem is not actually about self-discipline. The reason we default to what we've always done and then beat ourselves up about it afterward is that we're repeating emotional patterns. To interrupt emotional patterns, we need to find out what our emotions are tempting us to do and consider what wise action we could take. Instead of immediately reacting to difficult emotions, we can pause and ask, *What's actually the best thing for me to do in this moment?*

In other words, we don't lack willpower. We lack awareness.

When we talk about awareness, we mean being tuned in to our specific stressors, thoughts, emotions, and learned responses to difficult emotions. Understanding the pattern is the first step in interrupting it. And once you interrupt patterns, you can stop shaming yourself for unwanted behavior. Instead, you can take wise actions that move you closer to your goals.

There's a reason we repeat patterns and then shame ourselves for them: we don't have clarity on our patterns. Patterns we are blind to are patterns we repeat.

After years of observing emotional patterns that sabotage change, we created an awareness tool to help clients clearly visualize their patterns. We call it the *Negativity Loop*. The Negativity Loop is the pattern of stressors, thoughts, emotions, and actions that prompt someone to self-sabotage. If it sounds awful, that's because it is.

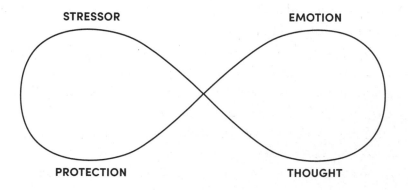

STRESSOR   EMOTION

PROTECTION   THOUGHT

To understand the implications of the Negativity Loop, let me (Neal) tell you how I discovered this pattern.

* * *

"Can you tell me about the last time you got angry?" Myron asked in one of our sessions.

"I don't get angry," I replied.

Myron looked me straight in the eyes. "Like, not at all?"

"Not at all."

We spent the rest of the session talking about how my father's anger issues produced in me an unhealthy relationship with emotions. If an emotion had a whiff of sadness, anger, or shame, I quickly packaged it up and sent it into the deep recesses of my being.

As we talked, Myron noticed a pattern: whenever I wanted to avoid a negative emotion, I did something to distract myself and make myself feel better. My common vice was posting on social media. If I felt like an impostor in my business (which was often), the deep shame pushed me to publish a success story about myself. This made me feel better in the moment because it "proved" that I mattered and that I was worthy of love—even if it was just through pixels on a screen.

"So whenever you feel shame, you overidentify with this image of success you've crafted through your work?" Myron said.

My eyes drifted to the ceiling, as if the answer were floating by the fluorescent lights. "I guess you're right."

"But this overidentification is what's making you feel like you're not good at relationships," Myron continued. "Because no one knows the real you—the person behind the image. It sounds like Carly doesn't even know the you behind the curtain."

This revelation was uncomfortable, but it rang true. The puzzle pieces were starting to fit together.

When I got back home that day, I pulled out some paper and drew up all the destructive patterns I was caught in. As I looked at what I'd written, it was obvious that these patterns weren't taking me anywhere; they were never-ending loops.

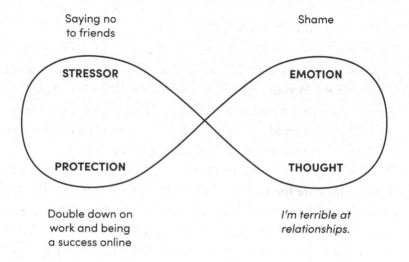

I say no to hanging out with my friends because I want to build my business . . .

I think I'm terrible at relationships . . .

I feel shame . . .

Instead of leaning in to the painful emotion and finding out what I could learn from it, I jumped to the fastest relief, the thing I knew would make me feel better: pretending I was a massive success through my social media posts. I was trying to convince myself and my friends that my success justified my lack of availability. This forfeiture of intimacy and vulnerability further distanced me from my friends.

The pattern kept repeating. Before I even realized what was happening, I let some of my best friendships wither away to nothing.

To make a positive change in this area of my life, I didn't just need to try harder or exert more willpower. In order to stop sabotaging my relationships, I needed to understand the emotions that led to this cycle.

I needed to get clear on my Negativity Loop before I could break it.

WHAT CAUSES UNHAPPINESS?

Here's how the Negativity Loop works. First, we encounter a stressor. A stressor is a circumstance that causes tension. You can probably think of ten stressors in your day right now. The baby is crying, you're late to work, you just got a big bill, you need to have a hard conversation. Stressors are all around us, and in most cases we have no control over when or how they come up. Stressors love to surprise us.

Most people make the mistake of believing their unfavorable circumstances are the source of their unhappiness. It's easy to point fingers at our stressors and blame them for our negative emotions. But according to a recent study, only 10 percent of our happiness is determined by our circumstances. Yes, you read that correctly: only 10 percent. The even bigger surprise is that a whopping 40 percent of our overall happiness is determined by our thoughts and actions. (The remaining 50 percent is determined by our genetics, which isn't as hopeless as it sounds, since we can change the way our genes are expressed.)[3] To put it differently, it's not our stressors that determine our unhappiness but our response to them—namely, our thoughts. Our thoughts assign meaning to an event and determine how we'll respond to it emotionally.

After we encounter a stressor, we have a thought. It could be anything from *This day is ruined* to *I'm a failure*.

The negative thoughts that run in the background of our minds are fueled by false scripts—the lies we believe about where we'll find happiness (more on this in the next chapter). For example, if you have a false script that you can't be happy unless you're in a romantic relationship, then you'll believe you aren't worthy unless you're dating someone. If you experience the stressor of a breakup, the thought that powers your Negativity Loop might be *I'm not worth loving*. Or if you have a false script that says more money will make you happy, then the stressor of a low-paying job might fill you with shame and fear.

Our negative thoughts produce negative emotions—often shame, guilt, or fear. When we experience negative emotions, it's important to understand that nothing is wrong with us. These painful emotions can often work like a yield sign, signaling us to slow down and exercise caution. The key is to acknowledge our painful emotions rather than look for the exits.

When we have a poor relationship with our emotions, we seek an escape or a protection to help us feel better in the moment. We use a protection to play it safe, but in most cases, it's just a way to run away from the pain. Examples of protections include overworking, procrastinating, bingeing on Netflix, drinking, complaining, obsessively cleaning the house, or shopping. The behavior may be different for each person, but the motivation is the same: to do whatever it takes to feel better and escape pain.

We keep going back to the same protections because they feel good in the moment. As crazy as it sounds, part of us doesn't want to break our patterns and negative beliefs because they give us short-term benefits. Psychologists call these "secondary gains"—the psychological benefits we receive from pain.[4] For example, there's a payoff in playing the victim because people rush to your side. Or you might enjoy relational drama because of the secondary gain of gossiping about it with others.

The more we repeat our patterns, the more they compound. Repeated thoughts become cemented beliefs, which produce knee-jerk emotional reactions. The more we escape our emotions with a protection, the more difficult it is to confront the source of our pain. So the next time we experience a stressor, it produces the same thought and the same emotion, except this time it's bigger. If we keep avoiding our

The more we

repeat our patterns,

the more they compound.

emotions, we'll need greater protections to help us jump out of our painful experience. The pattern repeats, and over time, it grows into a sense of hopelessness.

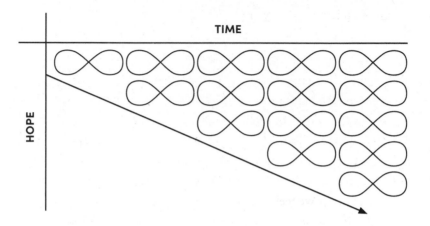

This pattern will continue unless we do something to stop it.

This is what happened to my (Neal's) friend James, who struggled with the decision to buy a house. His fear of not feeling capable with money pushed him to avoid thinking about finances altogether. But because he wasn't paying attention to this area of his life, his stressors got worse over time. This unhealthy relationship with money compounded. He wasn't taking care of himself financially, and it was hurting his family.

A similar scenario can play out in just about any area of life. Maybe you are afraid of failing on a big project, so you procrastinate on starting it. This just amplifies your anxiety because now you have more work to run away from—and less time to do it. Or maybe you feel like you're a bad partner when you're arguing with your spouse. In an attempt to protect yourself from this shame, you practice the same protection response of yelling and getting defensive. But this only further sabotages your relationship.

Starting from joy is the intentional practice of breaking patterns of shame, guilt, and fear. It's about confronting pain, sitting with it, and pursuing the wise actions that move us forward.

PLAY-IT-SAFE RESPONSES

After years of working with people to deconstruct their loops, Carly and I began to notice a pattern. Most protection responses fall into three categories: bingeing, avoidance, and rage.

With the binge response, we deal with hard emotions by overdoing something. It's often brought on when we feel fearful, restricted, or overwhelmed. Bingeing behaviors include overworking, overeating, overexercising, overspending, and overthinking. We fear we won't get our work done, so we overwork. Or we feel restricted in our eating, so we binge eat. Or we feel anxious and fearful, so we binge our thoughts by diving into worry. We blow past healthy limits in an attempt to feel better.

The avoidance response is when we deal with difficult emotions by withdrawing. It's often brought on when we feel like we don't have the resources to handle our stressors or we don't want to do the work of paying attention to our emotions. Avoidance behaviors include procrastinating, watching TV for hours on end, isolating, buying a plane ticket to go on vacation when work is hard, burying emotions, and just shutting down. Sometimes it's good to disconnect from the world, but when we consistently use avoidance to run from hard things and ignore the reality of our circumstances, our Negativity Loops deepen.

The rage response is when we deal with hard emotions by dispelling the negative energy at someone else. It's often brought on when we want to avoid personal ownership or when we feel triggered by shame. Examples of a rage protection response include blaming, complaining, criticizing, becoming defensive, venting on Facebook, blowing up at a significant other, and letting anger get out of control. Anger in itself is not a bad emotion. But a rage response is like taking a bottle of soda and shaking it up: what comes out is often too much. And an untamed rage protection response can destroy relationships.

These common protection responses are ways we play it safe, but ultimately they hold us back from positive change.

BREAKING THE PATTERN

After helping dozens of clients work through their bingeing, avoidance, and rage protection responses, we've found specific wise actions that can break Negativity Loops. Here are the wise actions that interrupt each protection response:

- bingeing → boundaries
- avoidance → attention
- rage → reconnection

Let's take a deeper look at these actions.

From Bingeing to Boundaries

My (Carly's) client Brenda came to me with a surprising announcement.

"Carly," she began. "I'm an alcoholic."

"What makes you think that?" I asked.

"Because I drink too much."

I'd been working with Brenda long enough to know there was no addiction involved. She wasn't dealing with alcoholism; she was using alcohol to numb the stress of her daily life. It was a protection response of overdrinking.

"What are you afraid of?" I asked her.

Her response was immediate. "I'm afraid I won't be able to control myself with drinking. Should I get rid of all the alcohol in my house?"

Conventional wisdom would suggest that going cold turkey would be the right next step. But I knew this wouldn't work for Brenda. Something interesting happens when a person is told they can't do something: the behavior becomes more enticing. This is called the forbidden-fruit effect. When we're forced to avoid something, our thoughts about it increase. This is often the case with clients who are on restrictive diets. If they're forced to follow strict rules about what foods to eat and what foods to avoid, they're more likely to binge on what they're trying to avoid.

Instead of recommending that Brenda eliminate all alcohol, I suggested another idea. "What if you didn't cut out alcohol entirely but put some limits around your drinking?"

She looked puzzled. "Limits?"

"Yeah, like you only drink on weekends or you don't drink more than one glass of wine a day."

People who have binge protection responses tend to live in the extremes. They either overdo everything or seek to cut everything out. There's little in between. This is why boundaries are beneficial—they help you establish safe guidelines for living in the gray areas, between overdoing things and avoiding things altogether.

This simple suggestion helped Brenda curb her use of alcohol as a way to numb her stress. When life felt heavy and hard, her boundaries allowed her to stop reaching for the glass every time.

Boundaries are simply about setting limits for yourself. If your tendency is to overspend when you experience a stressor, consider setting a boundary to follow a spending plan or to shop only when you need something. If you're known to overwork, set a boundary for when you'll end work for the day, and then establish some barriers so you're not tempted to work at home (e.g., keeping your computer in the closet, turning off your phone, etc.). If you tend to overexercise, establish a limit, such as exercising for only a certain amount of time, paying attention to which muscle groups are sore, and avoiding anything that might push them too far.

Setting limits when you're prone to overdoing behaviors is a wise action to take in your quest for joy and change.

From Avoidance to Attention

The other day, I (Neal) received an email from a reader that said, "I had no idea that budgeting could be a form of self-care. My mind is blown!" This reader explained that she had a lot of debt, but in an attempt to prevent herself from feeling pain, she avoided creating a plan to pay down that debt. Instead, she lived in ignorance of her debt and continued spending money on her credit cards. As a result, her debt grew, and this Negativity Loop compounded, with some real-world consequences.

When she read my *Joyletter** about making a plan for money and giving attention to it, everything changed for her. She saw that budgeting could give her hope for a better financial future. She found meaning in setting a budget, and this mindset shift helped her find pleasure in managing her finances. She's no longer fighting her willpower when she sits down to work on her budget. Instead, she sees it as a form of self-care—a way to tend to her emotional *and* financial health.

Our brains can trick us into running away from the source of our pain. This is good when you're trying to escape a tiger that wants to eat you, but it's bad when you're avoiding your bank account and budget. Instead of ignoring the source of our stress, we need to pay attention to it. If your protection response is to ignore how much you're spending, you can take a couple of minutes to look at your budget before making a purchase. Or if your protection response is procrastination, you can take a little time each evening to look at your schedule for the next day and write down your priorities.

Instead of avoiding our stressors, we can direct attention to them and give them the space they need.

From Rage to Reconnection

Brené Brown defines blame as the discharge of discomfort and pain. When something bad happens, we look for someone else to take

---

* Only the best online newsletter, which you can find at enjoycowellness.com/story/.

ownership. Blame has an inverse relationship with accountability. When we blame, we're not actually holding someone accountable; we're more interested in helping ourselves feel better.[5]

Blame is a rage response that corrodes our relationships. When we experience a negative emotion and blame someone else, we end up driving a wedge in the relationship. We use the incident as justification for our rage.

Someone once told me (Neal) that rage is showing up bigger than the fear inside you. I would edit that and say that rage is showing up bigger than the shame, guilt, and fear inside you. But what if we didn't have to show up bigger? What if we could assume a gentle and lowly heart, like that of Christ?[6] What if we didn't need to seek retribution but instead humbled ourselves? It was out of humility that Jesus healed the world.[7] We can learn something from that example.

When we feel tempted to rage, the wise action is to reconnect.** When we think someone has done us wrong, it's second nature to want to explode at them. But giving in to a rage response only compounds our Negativity Loop and destroys our relationships. Not only that, but rage doesn't hold a person accountable. To reconnect in the midst of painful emotions, simply acknowledge that what the other person did made you feel [insert painful emotion]. You don't have to show up bigger; you don't have to make them pay. You just have to turn toward them instead of letting rage create a rift.

But reconnecting doesn't just mean reconnecting with others. It also means reconnecting with *yourself*. If something makes you angry and you're tempted to vent on social media, take a pause. Ask yourself, *What's the value underneath this anger? Why am I so upset about this?* Reconnect with what's under the surface, with what feels lost for you. As you identify the heart behind the action, you can advocate for yourself in healthier ways that actually address the pain. For instance,

---

** Note that reconnection is intended for healthy, safe relationships. For instance, it's not wise for an abuse victim to reconnect with their abuser without guidance and discernment.

if you feel defensive and you're tempted to blow up at your spouse, ask yourself, *What unwanted part of my identity am I protecting myself from?* Then you'll be able to talk to your spouse from a place of vulnerability and safety.

In a society where people hastily respond to discomfort and pain in maladaptive ways, it's possible to break the cycle. We can use uncomfortable emotions as signs to lead us to reconnect with ourselves and others. This act of care can not only heal our relationships but also bring light into a world marked by brokenness.

HOW THE LOOP PLAYS OUT IN REAL LIFE

I (Carly) help many clients identify their Negativity Loop and how it sabotages them. Here's an example from my client Jennifer, who struggled with hating her body.

- **Stressor:** going to the gym and comparing herself to everyone else
- **Thought:** *I don't belong here. I shouldn't be here.*
- **Emotion:** shame
- **Protection:** isolating and not engaging in healthy movement (avoidance)

This Negativity Loop had real-life consequences for Jennifer's health and her view of her body.

Here's a Negativity Loop from another client, Ryan, who struggled with finances:

- **Stressor:** a big bill
- **Thought:** *I can't stick to my budget.*
- **Emotion:** fear
- **Protection:** overspending (bingeing)

Notice how his protection stood in direct contrast to his long-term goal. When we're overwhelmed with hard emotions, our rational brain often succumbs to the weight.

The same was true for my client Nate, who struggled with agoraphobia. Here was his Negativity Loop:

- **Stressor:** leaving the house while tired
- **Thought:** *I'm too tired to go out. I might have a panic attack.*
- **Emotion:** fear and anxiety
- **Protection:** isolating, staying up late (avoidance)

The work Nate did with me to interrupt his patterns was intense. But he was willing to do it.

HOW TO INTERRUPT A NEGATIVITY LOOP

Nate didn't want to struggle with agoraphobia. He wanted to see his friends, go to college, and get a good job. He wanted to enjoy his life.

To build a life he enjoyed, he needed to identify his first goal. He decided he wanted to go to college in person. There were several hurdles in his way. Since he'd dropped out of high school, he had to get his GED and take a standardized test before he could apply to college. Not only did he have to take the exam, but he had to show up *in person*.

These were not unrealistic expectations. In my bones, I knew he could do this. But first we needed to address the elephant in the room: his anxiety. If he was going to stop isolating and staying up late in response to anxiety, he had to change his relationship with this emotion.

Nate had an avoidance protection response. The only way for him to interrupt his pattern was to pay attention to the emotion forcing his isolation and sit with it long enough to not run away.

I issued a challenge for Nate. The next time he was tempted to cancel his session with me, I encouraged him to take a moment to sit with the anxiety. He could still cancel his session, but with a caveat. If he canceled, he had to pay the cancellation fee and he had to express what was triggering his fear. Only then could he reschedule for later in the week.

The more he paid attention to his anxiety and how it was sabotaging his life, the more courageous he became in facing it. Instead of allowing his anxiety to rule, he gained power over it.

On the day of his GED exam, his heart was pounding as he pulled into the parking lot. He reminded himself that he'd already accomplished one win: parking his car. Now it was time to go all the way. He walked into the building, found the room, and took the exam.

And he passed.

He studied again—this time for the college entrance test. He parked his car at the testing site, walked into the room, and . . . passed again.

But he didn't stop there. As soon as he got the results, he sent in two college applications. Then he got a job to help pay for school. He would have to go to the job *in person*. Nate was a new person.

Shortly before Nate headed to his freshman year of college, he came into my office and we had the biggest party a fifty-minute therapy session would allow. I had his favorite snacks and drinks, and we even danced to music he'd produced himself.

As we threw our arms in the air, being silly and free, I was reminded that we all have this kind of potential within us. We might feel hopelessly bound to the patterns that compound our shame, guilt, and fear. But underneath the behaviors we struggle with are unaddressed patterns we can interrupt once we gain clarity about them. Then, like Nate, we can dance wild and free, celebrating our newfound freedom.

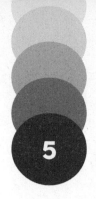

5 CHALLENGE FALSE SCRIPTS

Instead of believing joy comes after change,
challenge your scripts about where you will find joy.

After I (Carly) broke up with that boy I talked to my therapist about, I dragged myself across campus. My shoulders sagged, my eyes and face felt like they were being pulled to the ground, and I walked as if I had a heavy weight tied to my foot. I knew the boy wasn't good for me; I deserved more. But that didn't help my broken heart.

I stopped by the coffee shop in our campus library, hoping some caffeine would slap a smile on my face. As I picked up my drink, I recognized someone at a nearby table. He was a graduate student in the psychology program, and we'd crossed paths multiple times. I sat down next to him and gave him a slight smile. He could tell something was wrong.

"Are you okay?" he asked.

I hardly knew this man. But for some reason, I told him about the grief in my heart.

"I just broke up with my boyfriend."

I told him more of the story—how I knew this guy wasn't right for me and how I needed to move on. After several minutes of listening, he reached into his bag and pulled out a book.

"Here. This helped me when I was struggling with something similar."

The book cover screamed of an eighties design. That was the first thing I noticed as I held the thin volume in my hands. Then I noticed the title: *If Satan Can't Steal Your Joy.*

It was a bit cheesy for my taste. But in that moment, the phrase redirected me back to where I could actually find joy—in God.

"You're right!" I said so loudly that practically the entire coffee shop whipped around. "I shouldn't let Satan steal my joy!"

Obviously, the road to healing takes a lot more time and intentionality than a coffee-shop revelation. I had several months of therapy ahead of me, plus months of work on my own. But that cheesy title served as a reminder that joy can be stolen.

We have this conception of Satan as a tiny red devil with a pitchfork, laughing as he wreaks havoc on formerly happy people everywhere. I'm not sure Satan matches that image, but I do think he would like nothing more than to inch us away from where true joy is found. In C. S. Lewis's satire *The Screwtape Letters*, lead demon Screwtape is writing to younger demon Wormwood about how to lead people's hearts away from God. At the end of one letter, he encourages the young demon that the only thing that matters is "to edge the man away from the Light and out into the Nothing." He continues, "Indeed the safest road to Hell is the gradual one—the gentle slope, soft underfoot, without sudden turnings, without milestones, without signposts."[1]

This is how we lose joy: we become convinced that joy can be found somewhere else, off the road to heaven and on the subtle enticing off-road paths. We believe the lie that our hope can be found in something surface-level, such as a thin body, more money, the perfect spouse, or a dream job. We believe the lie that joy is a destination we have to find—one we arrive at only after putting ourselves through great pain. And we believe the lie that joy comes *after* the diet, the money, the wedding, or the career move.

That's the lie I bought into myself. I believed joy was on the other side of being in a relationship.

What we believe about where we find joy matters.

FINDING JOY FOR TODAY

Imagine this: You wake up feeling groggy and famished in the morning. You stumble out of bed, and the first thing you do is check your weight on the scale in your bathroom. You mumble discontentedly, get ready, and skip breakfast. At work, you grab something for lunch, but your thoughts are raging, shaming you for eating "so much." These restrictive habits follow you home, and you go back to bed hearing your stomach rumble.

Or picture this: You wake up and the first thought on your mind is work. You reach for your phone, scan your emails, and shoot off some replies. You rush through breakfast and head to the office. For hours, you pour yourself into your work, hoping that one day your boss will recognize your efforts and finally give you that promotion. By the time you get home, your family is already asleep. You collapse into bed, thinking about your unanswered emails.

We've been sold a false story about where we can find joy.

After we commit to the diet and lose the weight, *then* we'll find joy. After we hustle at work and get the promotion, *then* we'll find joy. The only problem is, joy is not a reward that comes after we work hard to fulfill some script. We shame, guilt, and scare ourselves to make up the gap between where we are now and where we believe we need to be to find joy. All the while, we miss finding the joy that's possible right now. Joy isn't a future destination; it's something we choose for *today*.

We've had our joy stolen by . . .

- cultural standards that say what size our bodies should be
- family expectations that are informed more by trauma than by truth
- social media that tells us what we "should" be or what we're missing out on
- self-help icons and influencers who sell self-centered change
- advertisers who capitalize on the gap between our desires and our reality
- our own expectations, which won't allow us to be happy out of fear of losing our motivation

Family expectations, cultural standards, unspoken norms, and the world of advertising all sell us a false script: that happiness is something we have to work for. It's a destination we'll arrive at *someday*, after we've reached our goal.

We're sold the story of "not being enough" so we'll invest in solutions that make us enough. We're bludgeoned with unattainable standards so our discontentment will lead us to spend more. As long as joy is a destination, there's more we have to do to get there.

These scripts invade our homes, too. They come in the form of judging glares and impossible expectations from family members. Often without intending to (or even realizing it), families pass on their flawed views about things like money, food, and relationships, and they teach us unhealthy ways of dealing with anxiety, stress, and negative emotions.

The truth is, you don't have to work hard for joy.

- You can have joy even if you don't lose the weight.
- You can have joy even if you don't make a certain amount of money.
- You can have joy even in your lackluster job.

- You can have joy even if you're not the perfect spouse or parent—and even if you don't *have* the perfect spouse or parent.
- You can have joy even if you're not in a committed relationship.
- You can have joy even if you're no longer young.
- You can have joy even if your health is compromised.

Just about everything in our world wants us to believe false scripts that counteract these truths. But following these false scripts has disastrous consequences—not just for our joy, but for our entire lives.

DO YOU BELIEVE A FALSE SCRIPT?

It's not always easy to tell if we're stuck in a false script. A person might think they're just being healthy, but too much of the real estate in their mind is consumed by this pursuit. They're constantly thinking about what to eat, evaluating every picture to determine whether they look fat, and obsessing over their workout regimen. Or they might think they're just trying to get out of debt, but their thoughts are consumed with this goal. They're afraid of spending money, constantly checking their budget, and endlessly worrying about their bottom line. False scripts have a way of disguising themselves as the right thing, when in reality they're just distracting us from what's most important.

Yes, it's important to prioritize our health. Yes, it's important to get out of debt. But these positive pursuits must be balanced with the right perspective or they become idols.

Idolatry isn't a popular word in our world, but the concept is all around us. An idol is anything that disproportionately captures our affections, anything we look to as the solution to our problems other than God. If we're honest with ourselves and humble enough to admit it, we often make idols out of our pursuits. Things like losing weight, getting out of debt, getting a promotion, or being in a relationship have captured our attention to such a degree that it's hard to believe anything else will satisfy us.

We continue to invest more time, energy, money, and attention into finding the solution that will get us across the finish line—to no avail. We put these idols on a pedestal until we're stressed, frustrated, and hopeless. This is always the result when we search for joy through external means instead of seeking the internal clarity that allows us to access joy today.

So how can we tell whether we're stuck in a false script?

The obvious sign that we're believing a false script is that we have an unhealthy emotional relationship with the part of life we're trying to change. If you believe you'll be happy when you reach a certain income level, you'll have an unhealthy relationship with money where you work past your limits to grow your wealth. If you believe you'll be happy after you reach a certain goal weight, you'll create a relationship with eating where you end up in an ongoing cycle of avoiding and bingeing certain foods. If you believe you're not a good Christian unless you read your Bible every day, you'll create an unhealthy relationship with your faith where you feel like you have to jump through religious hoops to please God. If you believe you have to avoid conflict in a relationship to be happy, you'll struggle to practice the intimacy that only comes from repair.

If you have an unhealthy emotional connection in an area of your life, chances are it can be traced back to a false script.

FIVE DIMENSIONS OF A HEALTHY EMOTIONAL RELATIONSHIP

After a few sessions with Myron, I (Neal) was hoping we would address why I was overworking. I knew why I was in therapy: I had an unhealthy relationship with work, which was affecting my happiness and joy. Yet after several sessions, we hadn't touched on my overworking habits. Finally, I brought it up.

"So why am I overworking?" I asked bluntly.

Myron cocked his head to the side. "You're overworking? Tell me more."

"Yes, I have an unhealthy relationship with work."

"And that's leading you to work more than you should?" Myron asked.

I paused. "Well, no. I take most Fridays off. And I only work until about 3:30 every day."

"That doesn't sound like overworking to me," Myron said.

I had a cookie-cutter idea of what it looked like to have an unhealthy relationship with work. It meant you either overworked or underworked. But Myron pointed out that my assumption was too simplistic. The reason I had an unhealthy relationship with work wasn't because I overworked; it was because I *overidentified* with work. In other words, I gained my value and worth from my professional pursuits.

When we think of unhealthy relationships, we tend to have a black-and-white view of what that looks like. We think an unhealthy relationship with money means overspending or underspending. We think an unhealthy relationship with our bodies means overexercising or never exercising. We think an unhealthy relationship with food means bingeing or going on a strict diet. But these assumptions don't fully capture what it means to have an unhealthy relationship.

Once Carly and I realized this, we knew something had to change.

For years Carly had been seeing clients who struggled with unhealthy emotional relationships. We wanted a way to help these clients identify what was tripping them up in a particular area, as well as how they could heal that relationship. During this time we learned about the work of therapist Pia Mellody and her five core skills for becoming a healthy, functioning adult after a challenging childhood. Based on Mellody's work, we developed the five dimensions of a healthy emotional relationship, which apply regardless of what your childhood was like.

Self-Esteem: I can find my worth and significance apart from this area of life.

Self-Protection: I can share myself without losing myself in this area of life.

Self-Awareness: I can accurately assess and share what's going on for me in this area of life.

Self-Care: I can take care of my needs and ask for what I need in this area of life.

Self-Control: I can limit myself in this area of life.[2]

If any of these dimensions are impacted, it means we have an unhealthy relationship with the aspect of life we're trying to change.

Self-Esteem

Self-esteem is about finding your worth outside the area of life you're trying to change.

This is how I (Neal) knew I had an unhealthy relationship with work. I overidentified with the successful image of my professional pursuits. Since I believed the false script that work was everything, I put my entire identity and sense of worth into my work.

The goal in healing self-esteem is believing you have unconditional worthiness—knowing you have worth and significance even if your circumstances don't change.

Self-Protection

Self-protection is about connecting with others while also protecting yourself in the area of life you're trying to change.

One of my (Carly's) clients, Robert, had an unhealthy relationship with alcohol, which was caused by the false script that alcohol would make him and his friends happy. Because he wanted to connect with his friends so much, he offered to buy them all drinks one evening. At the end of the night, he was stuck with a $2,000 tab. He didn't know how to connect with others while protecting himself.

Some people are too connected with others and have underdeveloped boundaries, while other people are too protective and have over-developed boundaries, leading them to be rigid and inflexible with their limits. We want to find the sweet spot between these two extremes.

The goal in the area of self-protection is having healthy boundaries, knowing you can connect with others while also protecting yourself.

Self-Awareness

Self-awareness is about knowing what's happening underneath the surface in the area you're trying to change.

We consistently convince ourselves that our needs and internal cues aren't right, which leads us to be disconnected from ourselves. I (Carly) had a client who had no idea how to tell if she was hungry or not. Because she believed a false script related to food—that eating little to no food would make her thin and happy—she shut herself off from her body's cues for hunger.

The goal in healing self-awareness is being able to accurately identify a problem so you can solve it and share real life with others.

Self-Care

Self-care is about taking care of your needs, relying on both your own resources and the help of others.

We are created to be relational people who need one another. But our false scripts lead us to either try to handle things all on our own or depend too much on other people. I (Carly) met with a couple who was struggling in their marriage. The husband was in debt and was consumed by shame about it. He believed a happy marriage didn't have money issues, so he kept his bank account separate from his wife's. His plan was to pay off his debt without her help, and he wouldn't let himself ask for or receive her help. The result was years of financial secrecy and an overwhelming burden.

On the other extreme, some people struggle to trust themselves. Their self-confidence erodes to the point that they delegate critical decisions for their lives to someone else. The reality is that we need a balance between the extremes of codependency and going it alone.

The goal in the area of self-care is practicing interdependence, knowing when to care for yourself and when to accept help.

Self-Control

Self-control is about reading the cues that it's time to stop and then being able to limit yourself.

It's true that too much of a good thing is a bad thing. If we have an unhealthy emotional relationship, we tend to swing between bingeing and avoidance. Someone who struggles with money might cut up their credit cards so they won't be tempted to overspend. Someone who struggles with overeating might purge their pantry of sweets to prevent themselves from binge eating.

The goal of healing self-control is to practice moderation, knowing you can keep things in balance without falling prey to binge cycles.

● ● ●

False scripts convince us that what we're trying to change is of utmost importance. While it's true that these changes are often good things, they were never meant to be the ultimate thing. God never created his gifts to be more important than our relationship with him. He created them for us to enjoy and to help us.[3]

In the show *Ted Lasso*, the all-around good guy and optimist Ted has a conversation with a therapist. As many people do when they're talking with therapists, he starts divulging old wounds and past battles. In this conversation, Ted shares that he was addicted to video games but instead of getting rid of them altogether, he decided not to deprive himself of something that brought him joy. Instead, he changed his relationship to the games.

This is what we're aiming for when we tackle false scripts and unhealthy relationships. Instead of depriving ourselves of good food, spending money, purposeful work, meaningful relationships, and other things that give us joy, we can change our relationship to them.

In order to do this work, however, we have to know where our scripts come from and how they entered our story.

WHERE FALSE SCRIPTS COME FROM

False scripts don't just appear out of thin air. They are part of everyone's story—something we learned at some point in our past. If we want to free ourselves from false scripts and enjoy life, we have to dig into our story and discover their origin.

False scripts predominantly come from four places.

False Scripts Can Come from Your Family

Our families of origin have a deep impact on our mental and emotional health. Even if you had the most God-honoring, loving, and successful parents in the world, it doesn't mean you're not affected by mistakes they've made. Most of my (Carly's) clients visit me because of their families. Perhaps their family has different views than they do. Or maybe their family hurt them. Or their family neglected their needs when they were a child, and they have unresolved bitterness against them.

Our parents have a disproportionate amount of influence on us. That's because when we're children, our parents are our primary authority figures. They provide the perspective and the tools for us to view the world and operate in it. We grow up in a particular family system with parents, siblings, and extended family who mold the way we show up in the world. This system can unintentionally teach us false scripts, and because these scripts soak into our brains at an early age, they can be particularly difficult to shake.

If you're struggling to see positive change in a particular area of your life—whether it's your work, your finances, or your health—consider what false scripts you might have learned from your family. Maybe at an early age you learned that women should find a man (or vice versa) to be happy, which leaves you longing to be in a relationship. Or maybe you learned that you can only be happy when your family is happy, which leaves you hustling to create the best life for your spouse and kids.

Dig into your family upbringing and explore if there are any false scripts that are holding you back from emotional health.

False Scripts Can Be Learned from Social Groups

As a therapist in Nashville, the capital of country music, I (Carly) sometimes see clients who are involved in celebrity circles. They gossip, stir up drama, and act like middle schoolers who randomly toss your friendship bracelet in the trash . . . you know, just like any other friend group.

One client met with me after becoming an outcast in her celebrity circle. One minute she was living the high life, and the next she was forgotten. Her group was petty enough to act as if they didn't know her when they saw her in public. She spent an exorbitant amount of effort trying to work her way back in, but this only isolated her further.

We grieved about how shaming this felt. But more important, we dug into the false scripts that this circle gave her—specifically, that she couldn't be happy unless she kept up with their social life.

Too often we surround ourselves with what Dr. Henry Cloud and Dr. John Townsend call "unsafe people." They create spaces that are marked by toxic negativity. They are defensive and self-righteous, and they lie more than most. They may present a facade of being good for you, but they influence you in the wrong direction.[4]

Because unsafe people bathe in negativity, they create a culture that attracts drama and pessimism. Our brains are drawn to negativity, which is what makes these scripts so compelling.[5] As we learn a negative way of thinking, false scripts begin to shape our lives. For instance, your friends might convince you that being a certain body size is the source of happiness. Or they might lead you to believe you have to have a certain type of job to be happy. As you scan your friend group, consider what messages you receive from them about where your worth comes from and what false scripts you may have internalized.

False Scripts Can Be Adopted from Culture and Media

When Carly and I first got married, we lived on a seminary campus nestled in the hills of the North Shore area in Massachusetts. It felt like a mystical place, hidden from the world like Wakanda or Themyscira (comic book fans will get it). This grace-filled bubble was the closest thing to the early church community I'd ever experienced.[6] People had gardens out back, we all shared everything, and we gathered together often. Best of all, everyone was poor like us.

Then we ventured out of our bubble into the real world. We got Netflix, met friends who didn't have jobs in ministry, and started our careers. That's when we realized how sheltered we'd been.

We were reminded what the real world is like. People have money, and they use that money to buy nice things. And ads follow you around, showing you those nice things so you'll want to buy them too. These messages convince you that you can't be happy without their product. Before you know it, your friend group becomes like an arms race of gathering more and more stuff.

We felt like aliens in this new world, like we didn't know how to fully "adult" now that we were out of the seminary bubble. Without even realizing it, we started embracing false scripts, such as the idea that money and things would make us happier.

In what ways has the broader culture influenced the story you believe about yourself and your life? Maybe the media you consume has taught you a script that steals your joy daily. To learn your story, look at the culture you grew up in or the culture you're in now and how it influences what you believe will bring you happiness.

False Scripts Can Be Forced on Us through Trauma

When we think of trauma, we imagine events like being assaulted, surviving a war, or getting in a serious accident. At least, that's what I (Neal) thought about trauma . . . until I talked with a therapist friend years ago. She said that a client experienced trauma from a haircut he got when he was a child. Trauma is anything that overwhelms our ability to cope with a stressful event.[7] Whether it's from a haircut or from being on the battlefield, trauma is a significant teacher when it comes to the scripts we believe. In this "little *t*" trauma (any trauma not considered to be catastrophic) with the haircut, the boy learned he couldn't trust anyone. His false script was that happiness came from taking care of things on his own (and giving himself haircuts).

This is the case to an even greater degree with "big *T*" trauma, the type of trauma that can lead to post-traumatic stress disorder. Trauma gets stuck in our bodies and replays in our minds as if the stressful event were happening in the present. We get triggered and instantly go back to the event, which disrupts our present joy.

Trauma often leads us to adopt the false script that our emotions are bad and that to be happy we must block out the pain. But this just results in the trauma getting stuck in our bodies and sabotaging our lives. Trauma sucks up unnecessary energy. To live a free and full life, we need to set our bodies free from that hostage-like situation.[8]

Trauma doesn't have to write the story of your life. If you feel that a trauma is affecting what you believe and how your body is responding to stress, we encourage you to visit a therapist. It's possible to take back control of your life, but only after processing that pain in a safe place. Consider what lies you might believe as a result of trauma, and bring them to your therapist if you need help sorting through these false scripts.

• • •

I (Neal) once believed that I could only be happy if I grew a successful business. I didn't know why I believed this until Myron probed into my history. My father was an entrepreneur whose business ventures often left us teetering on the edge of poverty. I grew up watching my mother work nights and days, and I wondered why my father's business didn't help us more.

When I became an adult, I had dreams just like my father did. But I wanted a different story, so I latched on to the false script that my worth and identity were tied to how successful my business was. I thought my success would validate my existence and prove that I mattered to the world. This false script was born out of the trauma of my family history.

The first step to challenging false scripts is to know where they come from.

- Does your false script come from your family of origin?
- Does your false script come from the people you spend the most time with?
- Does your false script come from your culture and the media you consume?
- Does your false script come from your trauma?

False scripts come from the world around us; they're never birthed out of our values. The reason these scripts shame, guilt, and scare us is because they pressure us to measure up to ideals outside our own purpose. The first step to being set free from their corruptive hold is to call out their origins.

Once we separate ourselves from the clutches of our false scripts, it's time to reconnect to our values.

RECONNECTING TO YOUR VALUES

My (Carly's) client Gina had a false script that told her she had to be dating or married to be happy. Underneath this false script was the fear that she was destined to be alone forever. With this devilish set of beliefs, she couldn't have joy where she was in life as long as she wasn't in a relationship.

It's true that our society makes it difficult to be single when all you want is to be in a relationship. Everywhere you turn, you're surrounded with the "happily ever after" false script and rom-coms that preach a message of finding "the one." I've counseled many women who long to find a companion in a world that is often lonely. But singleness doesn't bar you from experiencing joy.

I wanted to grab my client by the shoulders and tell her, "You are still worthy without a man in your life! You can still be happy!"

Of course, I didn't do this. Even if I had, she wouldn't have believed me. Instead, I helped her get curious about her emotions.

"What's underneath that fear?" I asked in one session.

Gina shot me a quizzical look. "What do you mean?"

"What is your fear trying to tell you about what you value?"

Gina thought about it for five seconds before a flash of recognition crossed her face. "That I value connection. I want to feel connected with people."

I leaned back in my chair. "Exactly. It sounds like you've let society define what connection means for you."

This was a light bulb moment for Gina. "You're absolutely right," she said. "My church culture growing up put extra value on finding a man. Somewhere along the way I internalized that message."

False scripts blind us to what we value. They swoop in and define what joy and success *should* mean for us instead of letting us create those definitions on our own. When we challenge false scripts, we reclaim what we value. Once we identify what our true values are, apart from the scripts we've picked up from family, friends, culture, and trauma, then we have to do the work of protecting our values.

When we challenge

false scripts,

we reclaim

what we value.

SETTING EMOTIONAL BOUNDARIES

False scripts are everywhere. For example, your family might praise thinness as a marker of success. Your social media might be filled with messages about the latest workout fad. The friends in your group might spend hundreds of dollars each outing. Your parents might continually criticize your occupation. Your relatives might ask you all the time if you're dating someone new. Or the people in your church might constantly shove the idea of being a "good Christian" in your face.

Even if you nail down what's most important to you, it's easy to fall back into old patterns. I (Carly) have many clients who come back to see me after the holidays because being with their families triggered their shaming patterns. So how can we protect ourselves from false scripts when we're in environments that tempt us to return to these scripts?

The solution is to create emotional boundaries.

Maybe you've heard about boundaries before and thought, *Oh, that sounds like something I need.* Yes, this is something we all need (and not just around the holidays). The problem is, people tend to think about boundaries in vague terms—as an idea that doesn't have much practical application. When managed correctly, however, boundaries are one of our most powerful tools for positive change.

I myself have transformed my life by exercising boundaries, especially around issues with my body. I used to go into tailspins whenever I encountered false scripts around weight loss. But my true value wasn't in my appearance. Rather, I valued feeling confident and positive about my body, and I could achieve that whether I lost weight or not. I protected my confidence and positivity around my body by setting boundaries for navigating environments that didn't practice this. For example, I unfollowed social media accounts that praised thinness and instead followed accounts that celebrated all body types. I also quietly excused myself from conversations that focused on losing weight in a shame-based manner.

Boundaries are the way we protect ourselves from false scripts.

With healthy boundaries in place, we can have a strategy for handling family dinners or dealing with a difficult boss or knowing what to do when a friend's conversation takes an unpleasant turn.

We've all heard about boundaries, but what are they, exactly? Cloud and Townsend define boundaries as the mental, physical, emotional, and spiritual property lines that "help us distinguish what is our responsibility and what isn't."[9] When we're hurt, it's often because someone has violated our boundary and put what we value at stake. When we build boundaries, we're able to protect what we value and stop false scripts from stealing our joy.

There's a common misconception about boundaries. My clients say things like, "Isn't it mean to set boundaries? It's too aggressive."

In reality, setting boundaries is the most loving thing we can do—not only for ourselves, but for others, too. Boundaries aren't about forcing someone to submit to what you want. If they were, then of course setting boundaries would be mean and confrontational. Instead, boundaries are about protecting your values. They're based on your actions, not anybody else's.

We live in a world that believes love means doing everything for someone else even when they have the power to do it themselves. But this robs them of realizing their potential and exercising their agency. True love doesn't enable; it empowers.

We see this modeled in the life of Jesus. In John 5, there's a man who can't walk who asks for help. Jesus could have healed him without asking him to do anything. Instead, Jesus heals him and then tells him to get up and walk. Part of the healing process involved an action on the man's part. Jesus often healed people in a way that invited them to claim responsibility. This is love—not doing everything for someone, but helping them realize what's theirs to own.

Maybe you've tried to set boundaries but struggled when other people didn't seem to respect what you put in place and kept crossing your boundary. This reflects another misconception. Boundaries are about what *you* choose to do, regardless of how anyone else responds. They represent *your* choices and *your* actions.

There are two parts to boundaries: the communication, where you let other people know clearly and kindly what your limits are, and the follow-through, where you consistently act on what you said you'd do.

It's the follow-through where most people get stuck. Have you ever said, "If you do that one more time, I'll . . ." and throw out an empty threat that you never actually do? When we do this, people learn that we don't actually mean what we say. No wonder it seems like people walk all over our boundaries; we've given them permission to do so.

The following strategies will help you set boundaries and protect your values in areas where false scripts reign.

Strategy #1: Filter

Imagine you're having a conversation with all the "popular" moms on the block. In the conversation, they trigger a false script: that to be a good mom, you have to be home with your kids 24-7. As a working mom, you feel annoyed by this. But here's the thing: you don't have to accept everything said in a conversation as truth.

Filtering is when you take what matches your values and leave the rest. For example, you could respond with something like this:

- "Yes, I value being present for my child too." This acknowledges the common ground in your values.
- "Yes, I can see that. Hey, let me step out for a minute." Then leave the conversation if it's too much.
- "Good for you, not for me." (This statement might be one you think to yourself rather than say aloud.)

Strategy #2: Connect and Redirect

Imagine you're at a family dinner and someone starts talking about their weight-loss journey. They're going on and on about how a particular diet will change everyone's life, and it's triggering your false script that you need to be thin to be happy.

The connect and redirect strategy is when you acknowledge someone and then change the topic. For example, you could say something like this:

- "We have different opinions, but I respect your take on that. How are your kids doing these days?"
- "I respect what you're doing to stay healthy. Did you see the game last night?"
- "It's good to be surrounded by people you love. Speaking of which, how is your family?"

Strategy #3: Share Your Story

Imagine you're with a group of friends who believe that kids get the best education when they're in private schools. Your kids are happy in public schools, and you value having your kids there.

The strategy of sharing your story is when you communicate what you're learning or doing and use this as an open door to express what you value. For example, you might say something like this:

- "My family has chosen to do school another way. Can I share why?"
- "Actually, in my experience . . ."
- "I've learned recently that . . ."

Strategy #4: Deflecting Unwanted Comments or Advice

Let's say your family decides to give you unsolicited advice about finding a spouse. Uh-oh, what do you do? Their advice conflicts with what you value and triggers all sorts of false scripts about needing to be in a relationship to be happy. This is when you deflect comments and advice you didn't ask for. It could look like this:

- "That's between me and God."
- "I'm enjoying what I have in the present moment."
- "Thanks for sharing your concern, but that's a decision that's really up to me."

Strategy #5: Control Your Inputs

Your friends' updates on social media are triggering old false scripts around work and money. Many of them preach working past your limits to make more money, and you want to reject that script.

Controlling your inputs means choosing to engage the media that supports your values. It could look like this:

- unfollowing social media accounts that praise your false script
- following new accounts that support your values
- choosing not to watch something because of your values

You don't have to let false scripts take hold of you again. Boundaries allow you to protect the values that help you find joy today.

CREATE YOUR OWN DEFINITIONS

Myron showed me (Neal) that I had a pattern of trying to prove my worth.

- I wanted to prove to my family that I could take care of Carly and our future children.
- I wanted to prove to my friends that I was successful and worthy of love.
- I wanted to prove that I mattered in the world.

But this pressure to prove my worth was exactly what made my work feel like drudgery. I was trying to use my business as a vehicle to undo the shame I'd been carrying for most of my life. This pressure prompted me to work harder, which caused me to spiral further with any setback, until I eventually burned out.

After one of my sessions with Myron, I asked Carly, "Why do I feel the need to prove my worth with everything? Why do I feel like achievements are the only thing that will make me happy?"

Carly took a minute before answering. Then, as though a light bulb went off in her head, she responded, "It's because you've experienced 'never again' moments. There are events from your past that you never want to experience again, so you're willing to do anything to prevent them."

As soon as she said this, I knew this was my story.

I've had enough "failures" in life to prove I was broken in some way. My father overlooked me. My mom was hardworking and loving, but any time she was sad, I felt like it was my fault. At school and church, I was overshadowed by the popularity of my brothers. Instead of taking a chance to get to know me, most people put me in a box, assuming I was quiet and shy, an outcast and a foreigner, lost in my own world. For much of my life, with people consistently looking past me, I felt like a ghost.

It makes sense that I would become obsessed with crafting a fake me—a success story worth loving. I believed that being successful was the only way I could be happy, but that false script was burning me out.

My conversation with Carly became both a revelation and a call to action. I learned that I would never feel joy and success unless I was the one who defined what those things meant for me. It was time to create those definitions for myself. That was the first joyful step in breaking my patterns.

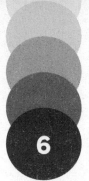

6 CALL OUT THE JUDGE

Instead of holding on to labels that inspire shame, guilt, and fear, get back to neutral.

After that session with my supervisor when I found myself burned out and exhausted, my (Carly's) mind started flipping through the pages of my life, looking back at how shame showed up in my story. When I broke up with my boyfriend in college and I saw my first therapist, I experienced a similar feeling of shame. In addition to those specific experiences with shame, I could see there was also a consistent thread: I had body shame.

When I was in my early twenties, I didn't listen to my body. I shamed it, called it "fat," and tried controlling it. It's no wonder I had problems trusting myself and changing my patterns. If I believed my body was bad, then I believed *I* was bad.

If I could solve my body shame, I reasoned, then perhaps the rest of the shame in my life would topple like dominoes. Then there would be no ceiling to the change I could achieve. So I sought out a nutritional therapist to help me heal this relationship with my body.

Kaitlyn had a calming presence about her. She was around my age, but the peace that flowed from her assured me she was full of wisdom. When I entered her office for our first session, I noticed the books displayed on her wall. She had titles that praised intuitive eating, health at every size, and body positivity.

I sat in a chair and sank into the soft fabric. After a few cordialities, Kaitlyn dug right in.

"Tell me your full history with food and your body," she said. "What did you learn about food and your body growing up?"

I told her that as a little girl, I learned that being overweight was an unwanted identity and that I should do everything in my power to avoid it. The problem was that even in a normal range for my height and weight, my family has beautiful curves and big bone structure in our genes. My body wanted to take a shorter and curvier natural shape that I was taught to avoid. This belief led to restrictive dieting, calorie counting, and ultimately overeating as a protection response to avoid the shame I felt. As a teenager, I already believed the worst about my body.

At this point in the story, I was crying. I imagined having a teenage daughter who believed such terrible things about the body she was given by God, and it tore me apart. No person should feel that way in their own skin.

Kaitlyn watched my tears fall and gave an empathetic nod. "So, early on, you learned your body was bad? That it shouldn't take the shape it naturally wanted to take?"

I wiped the tears from my eyes. "Yes. I spent so much of my life under that judgment. I want to fully love my body. I don't want to shame it or force it to change. I want to change my relationship with it so I can take care of it. That's why I'm here."

Kaitlyn smiled. "Then let's get to work."

THE PROBLEM WITH ABSOLUTES

How would you fill in these blanks?

- My body is _____.
- The food I eat is _____.
- My finances are _____.
- My work is _____.
- My relationships are _____.
- My dating life is _____.
- My age is _____.

Maybe you put words like *bad, terrible, awful,* or *hopeless* in these blanks. Or maybe you used words like *okay, great,* or *good* but act as if the opposite is true.

- If you believe your body is bad, you'll shame it.
- If you label the food you eat as terrible, you'll guilt yourself.
- If you feel your finances are hopeless, you'll live in fear about the future.

These judgments are oversimplifications of how the world works. Nothing's all bad or all good. Our minds like to trick us into viewing the world in all-or-nothing terms or as a series of absolutes, but these snap judgments aren't adequate for our complex reality. And these judgments only push us into behaviors that shut down our potential for positive change.

Our brains make snap judgments for a reason: as a survival tactic. The brain relies on speedy thinking to quickly steer us toward the direction of survival.[1] As a result, it loves certainty and sticking to what's familiar. Labeling something as right or wrong helps us use less energy in pursuit of survival. If one of our early ancestors saw a lion in the distance, their brain had to make a snap decision about

Any voice that uses
shame, guilt, and fear
to motivate is not
from God.

whether to engage the fight-or-flight response. It would quickly label the lion as a danger, creating an emotional response that would trigger an action (running away). In these crisis situations, there's no room for hesitation or uncertainty. If our brains didn't make snap decisions, we would die.

This is the gift of snap judgment—to protect us. The problem is, not everything outside our door is a lion. When we make judgments like "Fatty foods are bad," "Being married is good," or "Money equals success," they lead to more shame, guilt, and fear.

We all have a voice inside our head that makes these quick determinations. The good news is that once we recognize the voice, we can challenge it and move into the freedom and possibility of positive change.

THE JUDGE

Imagine a judge in a courtroom setting. This judge has one job: to render a verdict. He or she will pound a gavel, and the whole courtroom will weigh in. Then the judge has the final say over what will happen.

Now imagine this judge is in your head. But this judge isn't fair or just; rather, it's a voice of constant criticism. The inner-critic voice shames you, tells you what you're doing wrong, and leads you to self-sabotaging behaviors.

The Judge is the inner-critic voice that tells us what we should and shouldn't do. The Judge is trying to help you by labeling what's right and what's wrong, but there's one problem: the Judge has been overtaken by cultural expectations, by other people's opinions, and by our own experiences. In other words, the Judge has been poisoned by false scripts.

- If the Judge tells us we should exercise or else, we'll start from a place of fear.
- If the Judge tells us money is bad, we'll engage with money from a place of shame.

- If the Judge tells us fatty foods are evil, we'll feel guilty whenever we eat something we think we shouldn't eat.

But imagine if the Judge realized they'd been using the wrong rule book all along and began reorienting their verdicts based on the things that actually matter.

We believe it's possible to change the voice of the Judge. But no one will do this for us; we must take responsibility. As various labels come into our heads, we have the power to hold them in our hands and question them. *Is this actually true? Is this going to reap the fruit I want?*

We are conditioned to blindly follow the voice of the Judge in our heads. But any voice that uses shame, guilt, and fear to motivate is not from God. Instead, God uses love as a motivating factor. To quote the book of 1 John: "Love has no fear, because perfect love expels all fear. If we are afraid, it is for fear of punishment, and this shows that we have not fully experienced his perfect love."[2] When we learn to call out this voice, we can push back against the influence of toxic shame, guilt, and fear, and get back to pursuing positive change with joy.

WHY THE JUDGE'S LABELS DON'T WORK

I (Neal) was a good kid. I got good grades, never came home late, kept my room clean, and didn't put myself in compromising situations. I was mild mannered, spending the majority of my time dreaming up new stories and business ideas in my room. But for some reason, I believed there was something wrong with me and I was a bad kid. I explored this with Myron.

"So let me get this straight," Myron said comically. "You followed the rules, didn't get in trouble, went to youth group, and were pretty much a model kid. Yet during that time, you didn't feel like you were good?"

I chuckled. "Silly, I know."

"If you weren't good, then what were you?"

"Bad," I replied without hesitation.

I could see Myron rolling up his proverbial sleeves, ready to dig in. "Okay, let's talk about that."

Over the next forty minutes, I told Myron about my life growing up. After telling him everything—the highs and lows and the vulnerable, messy parts—he gave a straight response.

"It doesn't sound like you were bad," Myron finally said. "In fact, you sound like a really cool kid."

"Yes, but being myself never got me the love, respect, and belonging I wanted. I always had to be a caricature of myself."

"So being yourself was bad? Why couldn't you be good, too? Why is it all or nothing?"

Psychologists call the brain's tendency to think in absolutes *dichotomous thinking*. In our pursuit of positive change, this kind of thinking is often the source of our undoing.

In relationships, viewing your partner as all good or all bad disrupts intimacy because it prevents you from seeing them for who they truly are: *human*. If you see them as all good, you put pressure on them to live up to your expectations or risk falling from your pedestal. If you see them as all bad, you can never be a team with them. After all, who wants to partner up with an absolute villain?

When it comes to your health, seeing certain foods as good and other foods as bad leads to yo-yo dieting and binge-eating behaviors. It also sabotages our relationship with food, which is what we need to nourish our bodies.[3]

If you elevate your job to a place of utmost importance, you tether it too closely to your identity. If you see your job as a necessary evil, you stay stuck in a narrow perspective of what your role entails, and your contribution to your workplace decreases.

Seeing the world in absolutes limits our ability to move forward in a world full of gray.

GOOD VS. GOOD ENOUGH

The Judge tries to turn everything into a moral challenge. We're either good or bad, depending on if we behave in certain ways. When we view life this way, we end up derailing our quest for positive change through a phenomenon psychologists call moral licensing.

In a study about stereotypes and decision-making, a group of students were asked to rate obvious sexist statements. Many were quick to reject these statements. In another group, the statements were changed so they were less sexist. In these cases, students reluctantly agreed with the ambiguous but less sexist statements. Then the students were put into a hypothetical hiring situation, where they were asked to determine the suitability of potential candidates, both male and female. You'd think that the students who strongly disagreed with the sexist statements would choose the equally qualified woman, right? That's not what happened. Those students were more likely to favor the man than the students who had somewhat agreed to the less sexist statements.[4]

This study was repeated with racial prejudices, and the same pattern held up. What happened? Were these students just a bunch of hypocrites? Did their word mean nothing? The researchers discovered that the students who quickly rejected the sexist statements had established their moral credentials. This gave them license to trust their impulses and biases. These students felt like they'd done the right thing by denouncing the sexist statements. Now they had permission to do what they wanted. When it comes to right and wrong, good and bad, we just want to be good enough.

With moral licensing, our confidence about past good behavior makes us more susceptible to future bad behavior. When we think we're good enough, we feel freer to do something inconsistent with our values.

When we see the world in absolutes, we moralize behavior that isn't inherently right or wrong. *Exercise is good. Spending money is bad.*

Eating that cake is a sin. If you exercise and tell yourself you were "good" yesterday, you're less likely to exercise tomorrow. If you ate the "right" foods during the day, you may give yourself permission to eat "bad" foods later.

The curious part of moral licensing is that it leads us to self-sabotage and then makes us feel good about it. We "treat ourselves" and say we deserve it, but we're merely justifying why we're acting against the positive change we want. We're escaping pain by pursuing pleasure, but this pleasure is void of hope and meaning. In other words, it's not joy.

NOTICING THE VOICE OF THE JUDGE

Derek always told himself he would live a certain life. He would work in a faith-based organization, make a modest income to provide for his family, and dedicate his time outside his job to ministry. He would meet his family's needs, but at the bare minimum. He was afraid to make more money, even if it meant a more comfortable life for his family, because he thought making more money was evil.

The problem was, Derek was talented. *Really* talented. He was the unicorn of his workplace, running the team and getting things done, while the owners relied on him to carry out the responsibilities of the business. If you were to ask anyone at that company who was running the show, they would probably say Derek.

Derek knew he could (and probably should) be making closer to what the owners were making. His family would certainly enjoy the additional income. Yet Derek felt conflicted.

"I never imagined making that much," he told me (Carly) in our session together.

"But with all you're doing, it's what you deserve," I replied.

"Is it?"

Derek grew up close to the poverty line and heard a consistent message from his family about how much money he would make. When he became a Christian, the church reinforced this belief that it wasn't good to make too much; otherwise he would be a "lover of money," and that was an identity he didn't want. Even though he deserved a salary that was in line with his talents and contributions, he refused to ask for an increase in pay.

The voice of the Judge told him that having too much money was bad. His false script was that if he avoided money, he would be happy.

The goal of our time together was to take the emotional charge out of Derek's relationship with money. He labeled money as bad and was therefore afraid of it. He needed to come to a neutral space around money—to start viewing it as neither good nor bad, but just something that *is*. This is the goal no matter what area we're struggling with. Instead of seeing our work, our bodies, our relationships, our parenting, and our faith from an emotionally charged perspective, we need to reframe our approach so we can view them with neutrality. When these stressors no longer inspire shame, guilt, and fear, we can do the work of healing our relationships with them.

Over the course of my time with Derek, I taught him the concept of the Judge.

"As you approach your bosses to have a discussion about a raise, what if you called out that voice in your head that says having more money is bad?" I asked him. "When you hear that critical voice, quickly label it as the Judge so you can get back to what you know is best for you and your family."

Naming this voice isn't just a clever idea; it's a strategy for taming its influence. When we separate ourselves from our thoughts, we can create psychological distance from our internal voice and gain leverage. This process is known as cognitive defusion. Defusion—or separating ourselves from our thoughts—is known to decrease the believability of negative thoughts.[5] In other words, naming that inner voice helps us sort out which labels are false and not accept them as reality.

As Derek learned to call out the Judge's voice, he was able to separate himself from its corruptive influence. Eventually he mustered up enough courage to talk to his bosses. To his surprise, they were glad he asked for a raise, and they ended up giving him *more* than he requested. This wouldn't have happened if Derek hadn't learned how to call out the voice of the Judge and separate himself from it.

It can be difficult to notice the Judge's voice at first. The easiest way to recognize it is to pay attention to how your thoughts make you feel. If the labels in your head prompt you to feel shame, guilt, and fear, it's most likely the voice of your Judge. When you hear this voice, try gaining separation from it: *That's just my Judge speaking.* This will help you reattach to your purpose and move forward in joy.

RESPONDING IN KINDNESS

The Judge doesn't just place labels on our thoughts or behaviors. It is most insidious when it places judgments on *us*—telling us that we ourselves are bad.

The Judge spews negative self-talk that shames, scares, and guilts us, and ultimately disempowers us from achieving the change we want. When the Judge speaks harmful things about us, it's not enough to acknowledge it. We also have to counter this judgment with self-compassion and kindness. Otherwise we'll stay frozen in this critical judgment.

Sometimes people view self-compassion as being weak and going too easy on ourselves. But recent groundbreaking research shatters these misconceptions. One study reveals that people with high self-compassion are less critical of themselves, have less anxiety and depression, and enjoy greater life satisfaction and psychological health.[6] Another study shows that self-compassion buffers against negative self-feelings and protects a person from feeling overwhelmed by their emotions.[7]

By having a kind response to ourselves when negative events occur, we can protect ourselves from the sabotage of shame, guilt, and fear.

If you think kindness sounds weak, or if you think you'll never change if you're too easy on yourself, consider that kindness is a fruit of the Spirit.[8] In Galatians 5:22 the Greek word for kindness is *chrestotes*, which means "usefulness." In other words, kindness is not weakness but usefulness. Being kind to yourself is the most productive action you can take to achieve positive change.

A kind response in the face of the Judge could sound something like this:

- *I'm just learning.*
- *I made a simple mistake, that's all.*
- *I'm not as bad a person as the Judge wants me to believe.*
- *It's okay—this is not the end of the world.*

When you speak kind words to yourself, extending care and understanding, you are setting yourself up for the change you want.

A SOUND MIND

In Paul's second letter to Timothy, he reminded his young mentee that God didn't give us a spirit of fear but rather a spirit of power, love, and a sound mind.[9] What does it mean to have a "sound mind"? Some translations use "self-discipline" or "self-control" here. As Paul neared the end of his life, he encouraged Timothy to control his actions and make decisions that are driven by wisdom, not fear; by perspective, not emotional reactivity.

When we're motivated by shame, guilt, and fear, we forfeit a sound mind. We take actions that prioritize feeling better instead of moving forward. Once we get out of the clutches of our Judge and respond to ourselves with kindness, we're able to calm our mind. We can detach from our false scripts so we are able to think clearly about what we want to accomplish.

Know that the work of calling out the Judge is not a quick fix. Shaking off the Judge's labels is hard work. I (Carly) know because

I've been there. In my work with my nutritional therapist, I didn't immediately start loving my body. But Kaitlyn taught me how to show up ready to fight that inner critic. Getting back to a sound mind was what I needed to heal my relationship with my body and pursue the change I wanted.

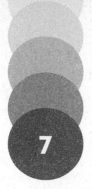

7 FIND YOUR JOYFUL PURPOSE

Instead of focusing on the pain of shame, guilt, and fear in your story, create a vision of the life you want.

After my first two sessions with Myron, I (Neal) still didn't understand why growing a business felt so heavy and hard. Every morning, I woke up feeling like my business was a ten-ton weight I was dragging with me. The fear of not getting clients crippled me with anxiety, and my shame over any setbacks riddled me with doubt. I didn't know if I wanted to continue with the business at all. It hadn't always felt this way. I remembered the days when I would practically jump out of bed with excitement for the workday ahead. I desperately wanted to go back to those times, when growing my business felt like play.

After my second session, Myron gave me some homework. He wanted me to record the ups and downs of my life on a horizontal timeline, from my birth until now. Then he had me weigh the significance of each moment using a numerical score from one to ten. On an 8.5-by-11-inch sheet of paper were moments of heartbreak, success, abuse, and painful lessons that carried me from my childhood to today.

Handing over the timeline to Myron felt like turning in an assignment to a teacher. He quickly perused it and then flipped the timeline around so I could see it.

"Point to when your business began to feel hard."

I didn't expect this, but the exact moment glared at me like a beacon. I pointed to it.

"There," I said.

Myron peeked at the page. "When you got married to Carly? Geez, don't tell her," he joked. "Why was that the moment your business got hard?"

"Everything got serious then," I said. "I had to care for my new family. I had no time to figure things out. I had to bring in the money or else."

Myron knew he'd hit on something. It was like he could sniff out the false script in my story.

"Is this why you feel so much pressure to grow your business? What do you fear will happen if you're not successful?"

I paused before answering. "My family would struggle like I did when I was a kid. I don't want my family to worry about finances. I don't want them to have the same struggles I had."

Myron nodded. The pieces were starting to come together.

WHAT ARE YOU RUNNING TOWARD?

We often feel the pressure to change something in our lives when we're trying to run from a painful part of our story. In my case, I (Neal) was running from my chaotic upbringing. I didn't want to repeat an unstable household for my family, so I put pressure on myself to get everything right in my business. When unexpected setbacks occurred, I spiraled in shame, fear, and anxiety. The added pressure of what these would mean for my family compounded my emotional responses, prompting me to self-sabotage.

Perhaps you've felt this way too.

Maybe you feel pressured to find a new job because you're running from a toxic workplace.

Or maybe you feel pressured to lose weight because you're running from the unhealthy patterns of your family.

Or maybe you feel pressured to read your Bible more because you're running from your old reputation or identity.

This kind of pressure makes change feel burdensome. It compounds our shame, guilt, and fear, making what should be enjoyable feel heavy and hard. As our difficult emotions increase, the only way we know to feel better is to sabotage the change we want.

Not only do false scripts present joy as a far-off destination, but they also ramp up the stakes when it comes to the circumstances we're trying to escape.

- When you lose the weight, you'll be happy. *And* if you don't lose the weight, you'll be like your family members who died too young.
- When you get more money, you'll be happy. *And* if you don't get more money, you'll doom your family to financial woes forever.
- When you find a new job, you'll be happy. *And* if you don't find a new job, you'll stay stuck in a dead-end, soul-sucking job the rest of your life.

Our false scripts fuel the emotional charge of what we're running from. But what if instead of running *from* something, we could run *toward* something?

In chapter 2 we looked at Jesus' parable about the two servants who, when given money by the master, went at once to invest it. They were running toward something with purpose and intention, and it resulted in more joy. The third servant, in contrast, was running from a reality he feared, and it ended in more fear. What if change is more about running toward our ideal life with purpose and intention rather than escaping a reality we fear?

When we take the pain from our false scripts and stories and turn it into inspiration and motivation, we find what we call the Joyful Purpose.

The Joyful Purpose is the authentic reason behind your desire to change—one that fills you with passion and joy. When you identify your Joyful Purpose and begin to feel the joy of this new perspective, false scripts start to lose their power. Instead of running from something out of shame, guilt, and fear, you can run toward a life that's in alignment with your values.

When pain is transformed into a powerful, compelling purpose, change feels less like a chore and more like a welcome opportunity for growth. We don't have to glue our eyes to the rearview mirror; we can keep our gaze ahead and intentionally craft a life that's in alignment with our values. When we find our true purpose, it's a clarifying force in our lives.

DON'T SETTLE FOR A SMALL STORY

There's a difference between a reaction and a response: the former is an impulse, while the latter is proactive. When we're proactive about the change we want, the process is fueled by joy. But too often the change we seek is a reaction to pain rather than a response to our values. As a result, our quest for positive change becomes tainted with disempowering emotions.

False scripts sell us relief from pain. In following their promptings, we live in a reactionary state, only focused on getting out of pain. This is how we might live a small story. Purpose, on the other hand, is about serving a larger mission, a purpose that's higher than ourselves. In her bestselling book *Grit*, Angela Duckworth defines *purpose* as "the intention to contribute to the well-being of others."[1] False scripts want us to escape pain for the sake of self-satisfaction, but this doesn't help change stick.

When we find

our true purpose,

it's a clarifying force

in our lives.

False scripts lead to shallow purposes, but it's not always easy to spot their deception since they're so ingrained in our way of thinking. For example, take a look at the beauty industry. One study found that advertisements for beauty-enhancing products such as lipstick, perfume, and eye shadow made women think more about themselves. Not only that, but these ads—even the ones without human models in them—lowered women's self-esteem.[2] To put it simply, the cultural noise around us prompts us to think about ourselves more, while at the same time making us think less of ourselves.

Here's the truth:

- Weight loss for personal happiness is not a big purpose.
- Getting a promotion so you can buy a new car is not an inspiring story.
- Finding a partner so you aren't lonely only works as a motivational story on the big screen.

Family, culture, and society at large will tell us these are important pursuits, and we should follow them as if they are our ultimate purpose. But I (Neal) want you to know: there's so much more out there for you—there can be a bigger purpose behind your desire for change. If you're pursuing positive change for a small reason, you're doing yourself—and those around you—a disservice. Your positive change journey can make the world a better place. And when you bring this reason out into the light, it will fuel your quest to make a difference.

Imagine if your health journey were about more than just losing weight. What if you wanted to improve your body's health so you could show up more fully for the people who look up to you and depend on your example? That's making the world a better place through your health journey.

Or imagine if your financial journey were about more than buying a new car or a dream home. What if you wanted to increase your wealth so you could have the margin to give generously and create jobs for people? That's making the world a better place through your financial journey.

Or imagine if finding a partner were about more than running from loneliness. What if you wanted to meet someone so the two of you could become a bigger force for the gospel together? That's making the world a better place through your relationships.

This is not to discount the pain in our stories or to minimize our desire for happiness. As John Piper says, "The longing to be happy is a universal human experience, and it is good, not sinful."[3] To seek happiness and relief from pain is part of being human. But false scripts take this natural desire and keep us focused on self-protection, self-satisfaction, and self-sufficiency, when there's so much more out there for us.

God doesn't want our pain to make us small. He equipped us to pursue stories bigger than ourselves and our own happiness. When we pursue a greater story with our positive-change journey, we'll find the passion and resilience that will give us lasting results.

So how can we pursue the Joyful Purpose that ignites our passion and changes our life?

IDENTIFYING YOUR JOYFUL PURPOSE

A Joyful Purpose has three elements: it must be authentic, important, and motivational. *Authentic* means the purpose isn't based on what culture and external influences say; it's something that has intrinsic buy-in from you. *Important* means there's something at stake if you don't live out this purpose. *Motivational* means the purpose gives you and others an emotion (mainly joy) that causes motion.

We remind clients of these elements by telling them to A.I.M. for a higher purpose.

- *The Authentic Question:* Why is this pursuit part of your story?

- *The Important Question:* Why does this pursuit matter for the world and the people around you?
- *The Motivational Question:* Why does this pursuit excite you?

Once we answer these three *why* questions, we can come to a deeper understanding of what's behind our pursuit of positive change. If these questions can't be answered, it's often a red flag that we're pursuing a false script about what will bring us a happy, meaningful life.

The Authentic Question

Why is this pursuit part of your story?

Maxine wanted a different life for herself. The generations before her had all died early, never getting to witness their grandchildren grow up. Maxine didn't want this to be her story. She wasn't a grandmother yet, but she could feel her bones aging and her body slowing down. She had a vision for a life where she was healthy and able to chase her grandchildren around the yard.

When Maxine told me (Carly) this, I choked up. "What a beautiful vision," I said.

With determination and a sparkle in her eye, she replied, "I'm going to do it, Carly. I'm going to get healthy."

What started out beautiful did not end that way. Over the next few sessions, I could see a burden slowly descending on Maxine. Her pursuit was no longer about getting healthy for her grandkids; it was about losing weight and fitting into a certain dress size. Her pursuit of positive change became an echo of the weight-loss industry, and she lost her connection to why she was pursuing this aspiration in the first place.

External noise can drown out our internal clarity. When this happens, we lose our passion. Shame, guilt, and fear enter our story as we see the gap between where we are and where we want to be.

But when we start to search for meaning in our life narrative, we can find a deeper reason for wanting to make a particular change.

When you consider why a pursuit is part of your story, can you think of a memory or an experience that motivates it? If so, it probably passes the authenticity test. It's internally motivated rather than shaped by external influences.

I (Neal) aspire to grow my family's finances. In some cases, such a desire could be motivated by our culture's view of wealth as a means to happiness. But that's not the reason behind this goal for me. Growing up, my family lived in the constant fear of not having enough money. They were always in survival mode, and this barred us from giving back to the world. I don't want finances to be the reason my own family can't be generous and pursue the things we care about.

If you're not able to answer this question with an experience or a story from your life, then ask yourself, "Where did this aspiration come from?" If it came from the standards of society or anywhere else, then take some time to find the authentic reason for wanting to pursue it.

The Important Question

Why does this pursuit matter for the world and the people around you?

False scripts urge us to pursue small, unimportant things, while a true purpose is larger than ourselves. If we were to drill down into why people want to lose weight, change jobs, or find a partner, the reason is often centered on personal happiness. This isn't bad, of course. But for purpose to have both passion and resiliency, it needs to be bigger than our own happiness.

Before I (Carly) started my private practice, I asked myself, *Why does this matter for the gospel?* I knew that if my business were just about escaping negative conditions or fulfilling my personal happiness, it would be doomed from the start. After all, building a business is not a happy experience 100 percent of the time. I needed to pursue something that mattered for others—something that would be a loss for others if I didn't pursue it.

As I pondered this question, I crafted my purpose: "I want to help people feel confident, secure, and free so they can realize that they were made in the image of God and that God longs to be in relationship with them."

I believe that God has created each of us with a holy longing—an innate desire to reach for something beyond ourselves. We want to belong to something higher and more fulfilling than merely living for ourselves. Above all, we want our contribution to matter. We want to feel that if we don't play our part within this bigger picture, something will be missing.

Here are some things to consider when answering this question:

- How would it affect your family if you achieved your aspiration?
- How would it affect your friends or your neighborhood?
- How would it affect your coworkers or your team?
- How would it affect your church community?
- How would it affect the global church?

When you determine how your aspiration affects more than just you, you'll experience a surge of meaning in your mission.

The Motivational Question

Why does this pursuit excite you?

A Joyful Purpose has to move you. If your purpose is motivational, it can move you to take action.

I (Neal) have talked with many entrepreneurs whose aspiration is to make money, but when they're asked what excites them about this pursuit, they have no answer. That's a clear sign they've bought into a false script. They're only pursuing this aspiration because they believe they should.

When purpose becomes detached from pleasure, we lose our passion. We give up before we experience breakthrough. When we find the motivational piece to our Joyful Purpose, however, we're able to excite not only ourselves but others, too.

Pursuing something for our personal happiness is not an inspirational story—it's not something others want to be part of. But if we're pursuing a bigger purpose and we're excited about it, others will want to join us. When we started Enjoyco, our friends were excited about its purpose and mission. This is how we knew we were on to something with our vision—it moved not only us, but others as well.

Here are some things to consider when answering this question:

- Does this aspiration fill you with joy?
- Does your joy and excitement about this pursuit spill out to others?

If you're able to answer these questions affirmatively, you likely have a Joyful Purpose.

JESUS ON PURPOSE

The idea of "finding your purpose" tends to feel like too much pressure for most people. The problem is that we imagine purpose as some lofty ethereal concept, when in reality it's an on-the-ground practice. While having a Joyful Purpose doesn't instantly make us happy or clarify every part of our lives, it does help us to live in alignment with our values.

The life of Jesus illustrated this kind of purpose. Even when he was a kid, he taught in the Temple. When his parents looked for him, he was surprised they didn't know where he was.[4] He was living out his purpose.

When Jesus was at Martha and Mary's house, Martha asked him to tell her sister, Mary, to help her with the preparation and hosting. Jesus gently rebuked Martha with this groundbreaking statement: "Few things are needed—or indeed only one."[5] Jesus reoriented Martha to the bigger purpose. He commended Mary for choosing to sit in his presence rather than busying herself with what was less essential. This is what it looks like to cut through the clutter and choose the most important thing—the one thing that aligns with our values. It's easy for us to be distracted by busyness and spread ourselves thin. It requires intentionality to let our true purpose illuminate what really matters, as Jesus and Mary did.

Just before he rose to heaven, Jesus gave his disciples (and us) a powerful call to action: to bring his Kingdom to earth.[6] This doesn't have to look the same for everyone, and it doesn't mean we all need to be in ministry. It means our Joyful Purpose—the calling God asks each of us to fulfill—can be part of the bigger picture of what he's doing in the world.

THE THIEF OF JOY

Sailboats.

That was my (Carly's) trigger word to signal to Neal and our doula that I needed help during labor and that they needed to make a decision. Needless to say, Neal and I were overprepared for the birth of our first child. We spent days practicing the labor experience with soundtracks, massages, mental preparation, and videos. Thankfully the labor was as smooth as it could be, and I never had to say "sailboats."

What I wasn't prepared for, however, was everything that followed the birth. I wasn't ready for the onslaught of the mom shame, guilt, and fear I experienced practically from the moment my son entered the world. Mom shame told me I wasn't good enough. Mom guilt told me I was doing things wrong. Mom fear convinced me that I was doing something that would ruin my child forever.

In those first few months, anxiety littered my mind. *Is he getting enough to eat? Is he doing enough tummy time? Is he sleeping enough? Am I ruining him forever by nursing him to sleep?* The loop of negative thoughts was endless.

Looking back, I can now see that there was a lot of good underneath those hard emotions. Part of the reason I was so worried was because I cared so much. I was trying desperately to do the "right" thing in a world full of uncertainties (not to mention that all this was happening in the midst of intense hormone fluctuations and sleep deprivation).

But these emotions also existed because of something that wasn't helpful—comparison. Comparison truly is the thief of joy. With social media influencers showing how they care for their babies and do everything "right," it can be difficult to sift through the information and figure out what's right for your child. And it's not just influencers who can prompt feelings of insecurity about motherhood. It's every friend and acquaintance who posts the highlight reel of their children's lives, leading you to have silly thoughts like, *Wow, it must be because they breastfed,* or *I can't believe their baby is sleeping through the night.* Comparison leads us to think we can be happy by following someone else's version of success rather than our own.

When Jude was three months old, we realized we needed to nail down our Joyful Purpose in parenting so we wouldn't be swayed by all the competing voices telling us what we needed to do to be the perfect parents. Here's what we decided on, based on our core beliefs: "Be emotionally present parents for Jude so he can grow up knowing he is loved by us and God."

This purpose does three things:

1. It gives me perspective when mom shame, guilt, and fear prompt me to get lost in the details (for example, it's not the end of the world if he's short on tummy time for the day).
2. It prevents me from being dragged down by comparison and reconnects me to the part of myself that cares.
3. It helps me filter my choices so I'm guided by my values instead of what other people say.

Either we can follow what we know is true and important or we can follow what others tell us is true and important. When we don't have clarity on the former, we default to the latter. Whatever area you're wrestling with, defining your Joyful Purpose will help you slice through comparison and reconnect to your values. It doesn't matter how you measure up to those around you; it only matters that you're living in alignment with what's most important to you.

PURPOSE IN THE FACE OF PAIN

It was an ordinary day in science class. The students were quiet, scribbling down notes as the teacher spoke. But one boy in the class was agitated. He wasn't bored, nor was he distracted. In fact, he couldn't rip his ears away from what the teacher was saying. The teacher's words were gnawing at him.

"Life is nothing more than a combustion process, a process of oxidation," the teacher said.

At this point, the boy had heard enough. He shot out of his chair and asked, "Sir, if this is so, then what can be the meaning of life?"[7]

The boy's name was Viktor Frankl, and he would spend much of his life pursuing the answer to this question. Some of his greatest revelations about meaning came from the time he spent in Nazi concentration camps. As he fought to survive, he observed how finding meaning in life allowed some people in the camp to endure longer than others. His book *Man's Search for Meaning* chronicles his journey of surviving the Holocaust and what he learned about meaning through that harrowing experience.

Purpose isn't just helpful when it comes to making changes in our lives; it also helps us get through the toughest circumstances. As a therapist, I (Carly) sit with people during some of the darkest times of their lives, when all hope and purpose seem lost. In these moments, people have the space to ask hard questions like "Why is this happening to me?" "How could God possibly want this for my life?" "How can I ever feel joy again?"***

In these conversations, my heart breaks with the heartbroken. It aches with the aching. I hear the longing for shalom in their cries—the desire for things to be right, the way God intended them. On this side of heaven, we often don't get the answers to these difficult questions. Pain and suffering are guaranteed in this life—they have been since the Fall in Genesis.

Because we live in an imperfect world, there sometimes isn't an answer to the *why* behind our pain. But there are some things we can be certain of in the face of pain: God offers comfort, peace, and his presence in our grief and suffering.[8]

Holding on to our Joyful Purpose in difficult circumstances doesn't erase our pain, but it can *transform* it. A larger purpose doesn't ignore the pain; it honors it.

When you feel stuck in depression, anxiety, grief, illness, or hard circumstances, your Joyful Purpose will not make you jump into action with enthusiasm or lightheartedness. But it can help you take wise steps that are full of purpose. It can be so easy to sit in hurt, anger, and denial and let these brew. Your Joyful Purpose, however, can transform your pain and help you move through it one small step at a time. At least, that's what it did for me when I needed it most.

GETTING THROUGH

For much of my (Carly's) story, I've struggled with shame and a lack of confidence. This was the case when I dumped the boy in college, when I started practicing therapy, and when I struggled to accept my body. Did I really believe I could be good enough? Did I have what it takes?

*** When we talk about a Joyful Purpose, we're referring to the motivation for pursuing positive change. We're not talking about the purpose that grounds you in the hardest circumstances, such as a cancer diagnosis or the loss of a loved one. However, a Joyful Purpose can help in these situations—just not in the same way.

Nothing, however, tested my confidence the way breastfeeding did in those early days of Jude's life. As a newborn, Jude struggled to latch. I heard the same brush-offs from the nurses and doctors: he wasn't interested or he was just too tired to eat. But in my gut, I knew something was wrong. My fears were confirmed after Jude lost too much weight in his first two months of life. He wasn't getting enough to eat because of severe oral ties.

Even under normal circumstances, this struggle would have been anxiety inducing for me. But with hormone fluctuations, a life-altering new role, and a lack of sleep, combined with genetics and a disposition that made me prone to anxiety, it was the perfect storm for postpartum anxiety. My anxiety elevated the real concern that Jude wasn't getting enough to eat to an irrational doomsday spiral. I tried with all my might to "take my thoughts captive" and change them. I desperately wanted to feel differently, to believe something else. But postpartum anxiety was a glitch that kept me looping.

In my desperation around breastfeeding, I needed my Joyful Purpose more than ever. When those anxiety spirals tempted me to fall into hopelessness, my Joyful Purpose grounded me. It reminded me that there was hope for what I was going through and that I didn't have to bear it alone.

From this groundedness, I was able to pause and ask myself: *What is one wise action I can take to keep my baby and myself safe?* The answer was simple: continue breastfeeding as our doctors and specialists recommended, and commit to doing physical therapy exercises and stretches for Jude at several points in the day. Sometimes an anxiety loop would tell me I needed to read every article and follow every rabbit trail about our situation, trying to find answers that weren't there. When I found myself in that spot, I would intentionally stop, tell Neal what was happening, and ask him to check something online for me and let me know if there was anything we actually needed to worry about. Sometimes the next wise step was to simply call the doom-and-gloom what it was and repeat to myself, *All I have to do is get through this night. God's mercies are new every morning.*

These small, wise actions kept me anchored to the truth: we were doing everything in our control, and now it was time to trust God to do the work of directing each next step.

Our Joyful Purpose doesn't put a happy facade over our pain. Rather, it points us in the direction of the life we want. Though our circumstances may still be heavy and our anxiety may still clamor for a place at the table, our Joyful Purpose cuts through the darkness and illuminates the way forward.

Neal's Joyful Purpose showed him what he was running toward. My Joyful Purpose helped me stay grounded and showed me the way through the shroud of uncertainty. For both of us, our purpose helped us reorient ourselves to joy.

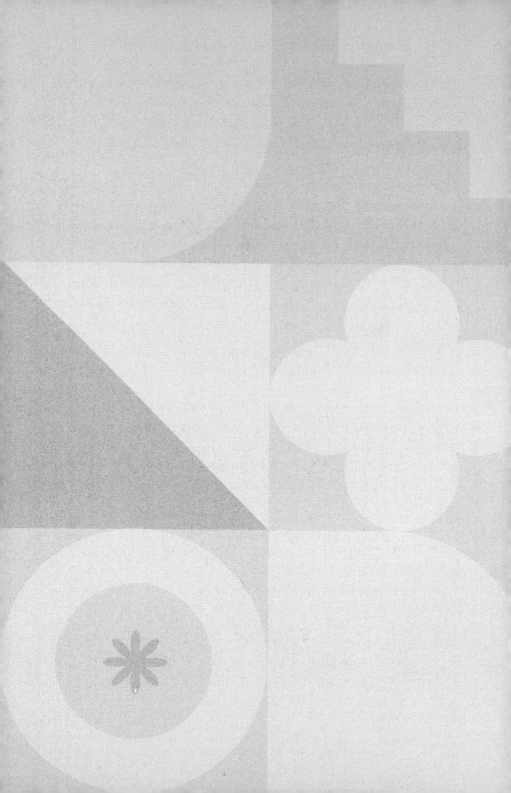

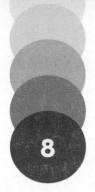

8 MAKE IT FUN

Instead of committing to the pain of positive change, make change an enjoyable experience.

One of the foundational principles at Enjoyco is that positive change should be a fun and enjoyable experience. Our studies in positive psychology show that when we enjoy healthy actions, we actually stick to them.

Here's an example from a client, Paige, who was struggling with going home for the holidays. Every time she was with her family, they had something to say about her life.

"Why are you still single?"

"Eat more—you're skin and bones!"

"One day you'll have a good job."

She could only get through this experience in a healthy way if she connected with her emotions, interrupted her loops, and developed boundaries to fight off her false scripts. But in the moment, these strategies can be difficult to implement—unless they're also fun.

So together we created Trigger Bingo. We took an empty bingo card and wrote in triggers Paige could expect back home.

- Comment about my weight/appearance
- Someone asking when I'm going to start having babies
- Aunt Mindy's opinionated politics talk
- Fight between family members
- Negative comment about my job status

The card wasn't filled with only triggers, however. Some squares were marked with coping skills.

- Saying, *Good for you, not for me* in my head (challenging a false script)
- Excusing myself when someone tries to talk about my relationship status (challenging a false script)
- Not grabbing a drink when I feel stressed at a party (interrupting the loop)
- Doing deep breathing when I feel triggered (being curious with emotions)

Paige started a group text with her friends who also faced challenges when they were with family for the holidays. When she got bingo, she let everyone in the group know.

When we make change fun, we create lasting results.

THE FREEDOM TO PLAY

"When was the last time you did something just for the fun of it?" Myron asked me (Neal).

I didn't know how to answer him. For as long as I could remember, I didn't do things just for fun. Everything in my life had a goal attached to it. I didn't write for pleasure; I did freelance writing to make extra money. I didn't build a business because I was passionate about an inspiring vision for change; I just needed to pay our bills. And when I spent time with friends, it wasn't out of joy; rather, I only said yes to opportunities that would open doors for me. Play was a relic of a long-forgotten childhood.

Myron pointed out that this lack of play was baggage from my upbringing. We unpacked moments when play and fun were ripped out from under me as a child. I recalled the time my mother got mad at me for giving an extra tip to the pizza guy. And the time my dad tried getting me to master several activities, including basketball, tennis, and engineering, so I could make my mark on the world. These fun activities quickly lost their appeal when they became something I had to do.

"Play is something we do when we feel safe," Myron said.

This idea made me imagine life as a big sandbox, where I had the freedom to move around the entire area and build whatever I wanted. But if there were a giant bug in a corner of the sandbox, I wouldn't feel safe playing in it. I'd limit my curiosity and fun to the farthest corner.

This is what happened in my childhood. I learned that it wasn't safe to play. I had to make money. I had to be important. I had to matter to the world. Those beliefs sabotaged my ability to let loose and play in this giant sandbox of life.

Over the years, I convinced myself that not playing was simply part of being an adult. What I didn't realize, however, was that we never outgrow our need to play. The desire to learn, grow, be curious, take risks, and go on adventures follows us into our adulthood. The question is whether we give ourselves permission to let down our barriers.

Author Greg McKeown defines play as "anything we do simply for the joy of doing [it] rather than as a means to an end."[1] After a childhood where I didn't feel safe to play, I stopped doing things simply out of joy. Every endeavor—my body, my food, my money, my work, my relationships—was controlled and had a goal attached to it.

As my emotional relationships in these areas healed, I began to rediscover the joy of play again.

- I felt free to say yes to all types of food, even if they weren't considered healthy.
- I felt free to make a fun purchase, even if it wasn't practical.
- I felt free to dedicate my work to things I cared about, even if it didn't bring in the most money or wasn't the best use of my time.
- I felt free to be myself in relationships, even if other people judged me.

When we put down our masks, stop performing and hustling, and know our own worthiness, we can feel safe to play, no matter our circumstances. The beauty of this is that when we give ourselves permission to play, we open ourselves to our greatest changes. If we allow play into our health, money, work, and relationships, it will be easier to create lasting change in these areas.

When you think about play, what comes to mind? Does this sound so disconnected from your current reality that you're not even sure what play might look like at this stage of your life? Or does it sound like a waste of time when what you really need to do is buckle down and dedicate yourself to making changes?

If you feel resistant to the message of play, pay attention to your story. Maybe you had parents who relentlessly told you to grow up and take things seriously. Or maybe tragedy and trauma forced you to let go of play too soon. Or maybe your church community pressured you to discount pleasure and fun in favor of a sober faith.

But here's the reality: it's okay to play, have fun, and enjoy your life. In fact, God created us to enjoy him.[2] And believe it or not, God enjoys *us*.[3] Enjoyment is a vital part of our spiritual life. And it's not just about enjoying God and experiencing his enjoyment of us. This joy is meant to have an outward expression as well. Like the believers who enjoyed fellowship with one another after the Holy Spirit came at Pentecost, we were designed to live out our joy in everyday life.[4]

Play is the best indicator of emotional health and well-being. It's the product of feeling safe and at ease in our own skin. When we intentionally add fun and play into positive change, we can enjoy moving forward and sticking to healthy actions. But in order to incorporate fun into our lives, we first need to understand what may be holding us back in this area.

HURDLES TO ENJOYING POSITIVE ACTIONS

Let's say you've tackled your false scripts around your body and health. You now know you don't need to be thin to be happy. And you've challenged your patterns by creating boundaries and determining wise actions for taking care of your body. Now you're at the point where the rubber meets the road. You want to go to the gym and move your body for the joy of it. And you know that if you can make going to the gym enjoyable, you'll be able to implement everything you've learned and build a healthy, happy life. But there's just one problem: you're not sure how to view going to the gym as an enjoyable endeavor.

If this is you, you're not alone. Whether you're trying to save money or finish a work project or date only emotionally healthy individuals, the right step often seems contradictory to fun. It's more fun to watch the next episode of a Netflix show than go for a run. It's more fun to spend money than save it. Why does positive action often seem boring or difficult?

There are three hurdles that stop us from enjoying positive actions.

1. We view positive actions as work.

You want to go to the gym, but you don't. What's getting in the way? Is it your lack of motivation, time, or energy? A recent study by the University of British Columbia found the culprit: it's your brain.

Simply put, your brain wants you to stay sedentary to conserve energy.[5] The brain is a survival machine. It works to keep you alive, and one of its most effective strategies in doing so is conserving energy. If exercise is work to you, your brain will try hard to avoid it. This goes for any self-care activity.

When we approach positive actions, we often start from a place of pain. We begrudgingly say we "have to" go to the gym or we "should" save our money. But starting from pain ensures that we will condition our brains to avoid a particular change rather than stick to it.

In another study, individuals were assigned a task. Those who viewed self-control activities as work were less likely to exercise self-control. But one thing changed people's responses in this experiment. When the word *fun* was included in the instructions, people showed more success with self-control.[6]

The way you view positive actions matters. If you view them as work—something that takes life out of you—your brain will push you to avoid it. But if you view it as fun, you'll experience more success at making the change stick.

2. We focus too much on delayed rewards.

One way we can enjoy positive change is through rewards. When there's a compelling reward attached to an activity, we tend to stick with it. But we often fail at setting the right kinds of rewards.

For instance, we think being physically healthy is the reward for exercising. Or we assume paying down debt is the reward for having a budget. Whenever we engage in positive change activities, we focus too much on the delayed reward. Here's the catch: our brains are conditioned to favor *immediate* rewards. And immediate rewards are more motivating than delayed rewards.[7]

Instead of going to the gym because you'll one day be healthier, you're more likely to go to the gym if there's an immediate reward connected to it, such as seeing a friend there or enjoying the exercise you do.

The same goes for money management. I (Carly) hate budgeting, whether it's for my business or my personal finances. But I knew that if I wanted to grow as a business owner, I had to practice financial awareness. It wasn't enough that my business finances would be cleaned up—that didn't motivate me to give my time and attention to my money in the moment. Instead, I made a monthly ritual of having a "Bountiful Blessings Brunch." On days when I engage my finances, I take myself on a date. I order my favorite brunch foods and drink endless refills of coffee while looking at my finances.

While long-term, delayed rewards will come eventually, we need the more immediate rewards of fun and enjoyment to help us stick to positive actions.

3. We dismiss the small actions.

We're conditioned to celebrate only the big steps we take toward change, and we see the little steps as things we should have done a long time ago. When we make small, pivotal decisions for our health, such as setting up an appointment with a doctor or a therapist or saying no to a bad date, we quickly dismiss them. But this view overlooks the fact that big feats are actually made of hundreds of small feats.

If we dismiss small wins on the way to the big win, it hurts our persistence and takes away opportunities for joy. Positive change becomes more fun when we call attention to these small victories.

The next time you take a step toward health, find a simple way to celebrate, whether it's high-fiving yourself, doing a little cheer, telling someone about the awesome thing you did, or just having a mini-party about it in your mind.

WAYS TO ENJOY POSITIVE ACTIONS

Once we identify what's holding us back from enjoying the next right action, we can take steps to counteract those challenges.

1. Look for Fun

The first hurdle to enjoying positive actions is viewing them as work. But positive actions don't have to be opposed to fun and enjoyment.

Yes, you can have fun moving your body.

Yes, you can have fun keeping a budget.

Yes, you can have fun at work.

Yes, you can have fun in your relationships.

This requires a simple shift in perspective. Instead of looking at the painful parts of an activity, we can look for the fun in it.

When was the last time you woke up and dreaded the day ahead? A recent study found that being afraid a day will be stressful actually makes the day more stressful. That's because such an attitude weakens our working memory, which plays a vital role in our concentration, focus, and productivity.[8] So when we start from a place of anxiety, our fears become a self-fulfilling prophecy.

When we're afraid change will be painful and stressful, we become less adept at the skills needed to make the changes we desire. What might it look like to approach change not as work but from a perspective of pleasure?

- Instead of thinking about how boring work is going to be, you could choose to focus on how nice it'll feel once you get your first task for the day done.
- Instead of thinking how awkward your date might be, you could choose to focus on how there might be potential with this person—and even if not, you'll get a great meal out of it.
- Instead of thinking about how stressful it will be to assert a boundary with your family, you could choose to focus on that exhilarating feeling that follows.

When we move toward positive change, there is a fun part to it. When we neglect this and view the activity as only painful, we damage our ability to create lasting change. But when we focus on the fun parts of the activity, our brain shifts. Choosing to highlight the fun parts of change will unlock our ability to stick with it.

Every morning, I (Neal) reflect on a question during my journaling routine: *How will I enjoy today?* Even if I'm not looking forward to the day, simply asking this question focuses my brain on what I am looking forward to. Instead of viewing the day from a place of anxiety, stress, or drudgery, I engage it on a deeper level.

Looking for fun means *have to* becomes *get to* and *should* becomes *want.* The next time you're faced with an opportunity for change, ask yourself, *What about this activity do I actually enjoy?* Or if you're simply anxious about the day ahead, ask yourself, *How will I enjoy today?* Choose to sit in that excitement instead of the drudgery, and your journey toward joy will have already begun.

2. Create a W.I.L.L.

The second hurdle to enjoying positive actions is focusing too much on delayed rewards. The payoff can't be in the future; it has to be immediate. The way we can counteract this mindset is to create a What I Love List (W.I.L.L.). A W.I.L.L. is a list of the people, places, activities, and foods you enjoy. This list helps you implement two key strategies in making change fun: reward substitution and temptation bundling.

REWARD SUBSTITUTION

Behavioral economist Dan Ariely had a problem. When he contracted hepatitis C and liver disease from a blood transfusion, he had to undergo painful treatment that involved injecting himself three times a week for a year and a half. If he did, there was a chance he wouldn't die from liver cirrhosis in the future. But the shots were unpleasant, and every time he gave himself one, he would get headaches and feel nauseous for the next sixteen hours.

As a behavioral economist, Ariely knew that we focus more on the present than on the future. The long-term reward of survival, though necessary, wasn't enough to make him go through such an intense experience three times a week. He had to make the experience more enjoyable in the short term.

He developed the concept of reward substitution—substituting an immediate reward for a delayed reward. Since he loved watching movies, on the days he had to inject himself, he selected several movies to watch. After giving himself an injection, he popped in a movie. Instead of focusing on the long-term benefit of the shots, he focused on the immediate reward that followed.[9]

A W.I.L.L. helps you reward yourself following a healthy action. If you enjoy a hot bath in the evening, you could make this an immediate follow-up after a workout. Or if you enjoy a certain coffee place, you could go there right after work to decompress from a stressful day.

The key to reward substitution is to shift your focus to an immediate reward rather than choosing a reward that's too far out in the future. When the reward immediately follows an activity, we enjoy it more.

TEMPTATION BUNDLING

Wharton professor Katherine Milkman loves to read books. It's one of the reasons she's learned so much about behavioral economics and historical figures, but she enjoys fiction too.

When Milkman struggled to go to the gym, she decided to use her love of books to her advantage. She only allowed herself to listen to *The Hunger Games* and others like it when she was exercising. She found that having something to look forward to while working out provided the extra incentive she needed. Now she goes to the gym consistently, five days a week.

Milkman named this concept "temptation bundling"—pairing something we don't want to do with something we do want to do.[10]

Reward substitution is about rewarding yourself immediately *after* the activity; temptation bundling is rewarding yourself *during* the activity.

This is something Neal and I did after the birth of Jude. When breastfeeding became a stressor, we knew we had to find a way to add joy into this necessary activity. So we chose a binge-worthy show we would only watch during late-night feeding sessions. We found that this made the time fly, and it stopped our minds from spinning in anxiety when we were concerned about him getting enough to eat.

Neal has done something similar with running. He loves to run, but he doesn't always have the motivation. So now when he goes on runs, he pops in his wireless headphones and uses the time to call friends. He pairs what he wants to do with a positive action.

* * *

When you're preparing for an activity that's a stressor, look for a way to make it fun. Refer to your W.I.L.L. and either pair something with it or reward yourself after the activity. A W.I.L.L. is a way to make positive change fun.

3. Make a Habit of Celebration

When I (Neal) met with Myron, I admitted that I struggled to celebrate anything good when it came to running my business. My achiever's spirit kept me pushing for the next milestone and didn't allow me to rest. For example, if I secured a new client, instead of celebrating what I'd achieved, I focused on how much further I had to go to get to where I wanted to be. This forced me to push harder. I dismissed the small feats I accomplished each day on the path to success because I believed success could only be counted and celebrated if it was something big. I also struggled with what Brené Brown calls "foreboding joy," or the inability to experience joy for fear that at any point, I would lose it.[11] I was constantly afraid that any success in my business would be short-lived, and I had to keep working to get to a stable point.

This habit of never celebrating my business ensured that I would form a negative relationship with it. If I couldn't celebrate the little things, I wouldn't be able to experience positive change.

I know I'm not alone in this. Celebration is often viewed as a risky endeavor. If we let loose and celebrate the little things, we fear we'll lose focus on our way to the big thing.

There are two problems at work here. First, we don't know the importance of celebration. Second, we don't know how to celebrate.

To solve the first problem, we need to recognize that without celebration, we don't have joy. If joy is the internal gladness inspired by hope, purpose, and delight, then celebration is the act of calling attention to hope. Imagine if you were running a marathon and no one on the sidelines cheered you on. Or imagine getting good grades as a kid and never having your parents call them out. After a while, you'd start wondering if forward progress was even worth it. Celebration focuses our attention on hope so we can find the pleasure to keep going.

The second problem is not knowing how to celebrate. We associate celebrations with elaborate parties or fancy dinners—something that takes a lot of effort to plan or execute. But we can celebrate the little things in little ways.

This is what we call the *celebration habit*. It's simple: whenever we experience something positive, we share it with someone we trust and have them respond enthusiastically. That's celebrating.

A study by researcher Nathaniel Lambert and his colleagues examined the implications of this habit. They conducted a series of five studies that explored the relationship between sharing positive experiences and positive affect (or a positive mood). The control group kept a gratitude journal but didn't share their experiences with anyone. The groups that shared their gratitude, however, experienced heightened positive emotion. The group that felt the most positive emotion was the one that shared their good news and received an enthusiastic response in return.[12]

Doesn't it thrill you when you tell good news to someone and they respond as if you just walked on the moon? Joy is heightened when it's shared, for both the speaker and the listener. Not only that, but happiness can spread up to three degrees of separation.[13] It turns out you can change a lot by just giving an enthusiastic response to good news.

Note that it's not enough to share your good news with just anyone. If you share your good news and the person doesn't respond with enthusiasm, it's a buzzkill to your joy. That's why it's important to make a habit of speaking good news to someone you trust.

When you capitalize on a positive event, you prolong the intensity of it. It's an act of savoring, which is a critical practice for joy. When you savor something, you seek to fully enjoy the experience. Capitalizing on positive events has been proven to increase intimacy between romantic partners, increase subjective well-being, boost self-esteem, and even decrease loneliness.[14] To put it simply, sharing your good news with people who respond enthusiastically is a great way to increase your joy.

Now the question is: What good news should we share?

In regard to positive change, we benefit from sharing any small step or positive feeling in our journey. When you feel good in the body you used to shame, you could simply say to someone you trust, "Hey, I feel great in my body today." When you look at your budget after a habit of avoidance, you could tell a friend, "Guess what? I looked at my money today." And when you feel positive about work, you could say, "I'm feeling great about my job today." The more you share positive news, the more joy you spread.

Aside from celebrating your good news and progress toward positive change, you could also celebrate *people*. When someone doesn't have joy, they navel-gaze. They stay stuck in their own perspective, which further spirals them into negativity. But all around us, people are doing hopeful actions. Even if you feel like you have nothing to celebrate for yourself, you can make an intentional effort to celebrate someone else. Call out the hope you see in them, and you'll light a spark of hope in yourself.

Joy is heightened

when it's shared.

People who are the most judgmental about others are also the most judgmental about themselves. They often feel like they have nothing to celebrate within themselves, and then they don't celebrate others, either. But if you reframe your brain to start celebrating the good in people, you'll learn to start celebrating yourself as well. People are worthy of celebration—including you.

When you have good news, share it. When you feel good, share it. When you make small progress, share it. And when someone delights you, share it. This is how you add play into your journey toward positive change.

MAKE FUN A PRIORITY

When we're lacking joy in our lives, fun gets put on the back burner. We sacrifice play for more serious matters, as though prioritizing play causes us to take our eyes off the ball. But the ability to play and let loose is actually a sign of health and emotional safety. As C. S. Lewis says, "Joy is the serious business of Heaven."[15] God's desire is for us to enjoy our lives.

Of course, play requires practice. At first, it takes a great deal of effort to rewire our actions and responses in the direction of joy. It doesn't come naturally to reframe events and start from joy. And when you start to build a celebration habit for the little things, it won't feel like you're doing anything significant at first.

But like the Negativity Loop, joy compounds over time. It continues to build until we start to feel it in all areas of life. As you practice play, joy seeps in everywhere.

This is how positive change becomes less about solving our inadequacies and more about making the world around us better. In God's refreshing sense of humor, changing the world is not the work of serious, strict-minded people; it's the work of those who feel safe to play.

PART TWO

Empowered
for Joy

9 ENJOY YOUR HEALTH

Ditch shame-based dieting and exercise.
Eat and exercise with enthusiasm.

One day, I (Carly) had a client named Daphne who was visiting me because she said she had a constant feeling of stress in her body. She didn't know how to describe it, but she could quickly pinpoint the symptoms. She was exhausted, had no energy to complete daily tasks, and struggled with feelings of sadness. Yet she reported that therapy was working. Her relationship with her husband was back on track, she felt like she was thriving at work, and she was meeting her goals. So where was all the stress coming from?

After several minutes of talking and trying to figure out what was happening, something clicked.

"When was the last time you ate?" I asked.

"Breakfast," she responded. She was my last appointment of the day, late in the evening.

"I don't think that's stress you're feeling. I think you're *hungry*."

"No, that's not it," she said, shaking her head.

I listed the symptoms of hunger and described the way hunger feels in the body. I talked not just about a growling stomach but an empty, gnawing feeling inside that reverberates up the chest and even in the throat, coupled with a "foggy brain."

Her eyes grew round. "I thought that was just stress and depression!"

Daphne wasn't struggling with an eating disorder in the customary way of thinking of it. But with her dieting, exercise, and disordered relationship with food, she wasn't feeding herself properly—so much so that she forgot what hunger felt like in the body. I literally had to teach her how to notice her hunger.

Maybe you can relate to some version of this. Have you ever rushed out the door and skipped breakfast, hoping your large coffee would do the trick until lunch? Or maybe you've glanced at yourself in a passing reflection, felt a surge of dissatisfaction, and thought, *I really need to get back to the gym.* Maybe you just went through a big life change and your body is still carrying the extra weight. If so, did you feel pressure to start a strict diet or exercise routine to achieve results? Can you identify with having this sort of relationship with your body?

If you've ever attempted to change how you look through drastic diet or exercise measures, you're not alone. An estimated 45 million Americans go on a diet each year. Not surprisingly, only 5 percent of these dieters are able to keep up with the change long-term.[1] Chances are, you're in the 95 percent of people who have tried dieting but couldn't maintain the results. Or maybe you're in the 5 percent who are seeing change, but you're afraid of what will happen once you're off your strict program.

We've seen clients who are all across the spectrum when it comes to this topic. I've heard everything, including statements like "I waited to apply until after I lost the baby weight, because fat girls don't get the job"; "If I looked prettier, maybe he would have stayed"; "No one wants the chubby guy"; and "I'm starving all the time, but it's worth it to reach my goal."

When we talk to people who are struggling in this area, we don't give them a solution for weight loss; we give them a solution for loving their bodies and taking care of them without the need for strict diets and workout programs. The idea isn't to love your body so you can lose weight. It's about loving your body just because you have an amazing body—made by God himself—that deserves to be respected and cared for.

If you're trying to make physical changes, your biggest need isn't to lose weight; it's to change your relationship with food, exercise, and your body. When you are free from body shame, punitive exercise, and fear of certain foods, you'll be able to embrace healthy actions that make a difference in your life, whether they result in losing weight or not.

The outcome could look like

- knowing you're loved and valued even if you don't lose weight
- feeling proud and confident in all the clothes you wear
- experiencing the joy of moving your body without strict, punitive exercise
- feeling free to eat any food and not fearing the loss of control with certain foods
- fighting off the false messages of the weight-loss industry

It's time to stop the cycle of repeating programs and constantly searching for results. Instead, you can adopt nourishing practices that fuel you to do the work God has for you in the world. Let's explore what it looks like to reclaim your joy in this area.

THE FALSE SCRIPT OF DIET CULTURE

Food fear, body shame, and punitive exercise are so normalized in our society that it can be difficult to tell when you're trapped in the joyless clutches of diet culture. You might think, *It's just a diet* or *I need to cut out these foods* or *This is how I care for my body*. It's not always easy to notice when your thoughts and emotions become unhealthy.

Here are some signs that indicate an unhealthy emotional relationship with food, body, and exercise, along with the dimension of healthy living they're impacting:

- You go harder at the gym because of what you ate. (self-esteem)
- You're only happy with yourself when you're at your goal weight. (self-esteem)
- You struggle with eating and drinking in social situations. (self-protection)
- You struggle with binge eating, under-eating, or emotional eating. (self-control)
- You can't tell when you're hungry. (self-awareness)
- You promise you'll be better tomorrow. (self-esteem)
- You don't know how to adequately exercise or feed yourself if you're not on a program. (self-care)
- You rely on others to make your food or you only order takeout. (self-care)
- You constantly take "working lunches" or eat on the go. (self-care)
- You push yourself at the gym even if you're hungry, sick, injured, or tired. (self-care)
- You restrict food during the week so you can have "cheat days" on the weekend. (self-control)
- You view some foods as good and other foods as bad. (self-awareness)
- You're afraid that people will judge you if they see what you eat. (self-protection)
- You avoid having sweets in the house for fear of losing control. (self-control)

- You tell yourself you're "being bad" when you reach for a treat, and you tell yourself you're "being good" when you eat healthy. (self-esteem)
- You use messages of grit, resilience, and mental toughness to suppress the needs of your body. (self-awareness)
- You rely on protein shakes, tasteless bars, coffee, and anything else that will help suppress your hunger. (self-awareness)
- Once you give yourself permission to go off your diet, you end up overeating. (self-control)
- You dress in clothes that hide your body shape. (self-esteem)
- You rely on others to hold you accountable to your eating habits. (self-care)

If any of these are true for you, don't fret—you're not alone. We've been duped by an industry that profits from our unhealthy relationship with food and our bodies.

For decades, the weight-loss industry has captivated people with the promise of finally feeling happy, confident, and successful. It's one of the sneakiest, most common false scripts out there: once you lose the weight, you'll be happy. People who believe this get stuck in going on endless diets, exercising past their limits, overthinking their food choices, and spending an inordinate amount of time, money, and energy on their appearance.

Diet culture not only steals our time, our money, and our health; it also steals our joy. Here's how registered dietitian, nutritionist, author, and podcast host Christy Harrison describes diet culture:

- Worships thinness and equates it to health and moral virtue (which makes people feel wrong if they can't shrink their bodies)
- Promotes weight loss as a means of attaining higher status (which is why people spend so much of their life trying to achieve thinness)

- Demonizes certain ways of eating while elevating others (which keeps people preoccupied with food)
- Oppresses people who don't match up with its supposed picture of health (which harms people with different body sizes and hurts both our psychological and physical health)[2]

The thing that strikes me (Neal) about Harrison's definition is how it uses terms like *worships* and *demonizes*. It gets at the idea that diet culture isn't just a way of thinking but a form of idolatry. Idolatry may be the sneakiest sin in our society because we often don't even realize we're doing it. Here's a simple definition: you know you've made an idol out of something when you worship an ideal and demonize anything that stands against it. Diet culture is a form of idolatry because it praises thinness and demonizes food and our bodies, all while distracting us from our Joyful Purpose.

It's hard to escape diet culture because it's all around us, from the clothes we buy to the television we watch. In 2020, the global weight-loss market was estimated to be a $262.9 billion dollar industry.[3] Wherever we look, we're inundated with images of the ideal body size, and we're constantly bombarded with the message that we must change our bodies in order to belong.

You might think that you're not dieting the way diet culture presents it. It's not about weight loss for you; it's about being healthy, and any weight loss is a bonus. This is what diet culture wants you to believe. Over the years, the industry has gotten smarter about diet culture. Younger generations don't want to diet the way their parents did, obsessing over programs, counting calories, and keeping track of points. Diet culture had to change if it wanted to stay relevant, so it became what Christy Harrison calls "the wellness diet."

The wellness diet is a disguise for diet culture that focuses on health and wellness instead of weight loss. But this is just a message change. To keep up with the wellness diet, you have to restrict food, eat the right things, and avoid the wrong things, and your body size is a measure for health. The wellness diet loves detoxes and "clean eating." It bans entire food groups and advocates strict exercise routines to help you become your "healthiest" self. In other words, it's diet culture with a makeover.[4]

Diet culture sabotages our health, our satisfaction, our faith, and our joy. It eats up our time and directs our attention toward lesser things. And it keeps us stuck in patterns that prevent us from experiencing what God wants for our lives.

Sometimes diet culture even infiltrates our faith communities. We're told that our bodies are a temple, which is a biblical concept,[5] but this is often misinterpreted to mean that we should choose the "right" foods or "good" foods, or that we should shed pounds that shouldn't be there. But the Bible speaks against categorically abstaining from certain foods, for everything God created is good and meant to be received with gratitude.[6] And God created us to pursue a higher mission than the surface-level goal of changing our bodies. He cares about our joy. Think about it: What if we traded the time, money, and emotional energy we spend on how we look for time with God? I wonder what kind of redemptive work we as the broader church could accomplish.

Diet culture damages all dimensions of healthy emotional living. It hurts our self-esteem by tying our worth to the food we eat and the shape of our bodies. It damages our self-protection by urging us to forgo healthy boundaries with food, especially in social settings. It encourages us to suppress our needs until we no longer know how to address them. It erodes our self-care by disempowering us in caring for our own needs. And it hurts our self-control by promoting unconscious binge-and-restrict cycles.

But the real cost is that we lose the ability to know our bodies and what they need, the way God intended.

When we believe the worst about our bodies and try to change them, or when we just refuse to pay attention to them, we lose

Diet culture damages all dimensions of healthy emotional living.

attunement. Attunement means listening to and acknowledging our body's needs. By forfeiting our judgment to external rules and guidelines for managing our eating and exercise, we drown out the internal voice that knows when we're hungry, when we're full, when we need to move, and when we need to rest.

Consider this: we were born with perfect attunement to our bodies. As babies, we had no trouble acknowledging our hunger and crying for food. We also had no problem letting our parents know we needed sleep. But as we got older and started to hear false messages about diet and exercise, we let the *shoulds* and *should nots* disrupt our natural attunement.

To challenge our patterns, we need to regain attunement and rebuild trust in our bodies (remember, trust is a gift of joy). Instead of treating our bodies as the villain, we need to respect them as the vessels God gave us to navigate the world. Instead of condemning the natural needs of our bodies, we need to realize that even Jesus attended to people's physical needs. In many instances, he fed people before he imparted his wisdom to them.[7] Instead of coasting through our day on autopilot or trying to push through as if we're robots, we need to recognize that God created us with limits. It's when we operate within those limits that we thrive as human beings.

So how can we enjoy eating and exercising? How can we eat without fearing weight gain? And how can we pursue a healthy life that's free of dieting and overexercising?

THE JOURNEY TO HEALING YOUR RELATIONSHIP

I (Carly) was getting ready for the day when I got a text from my client Audre, who had a session with me later that day. It read,

> Well, Carly, I just want to give you a heads-up about what we need to talk about today. I'll send you this message I got over the weekend, so I can process it with you . . .

I went on to read one of the worst breakup texts I've ever read, sent by her boyfriend:

> You have a beautiful personality, and I can't ignore we have so much in common. But I have to be honest, I just can't be with a woman if weight is an issue . . . Health is a value of mine, and I need to see that you're a woman who can follow through with her health goals. I'd like to reevaluate in three months, but for now, I just don't want a relationship.

That last line made me laugh—as if my client would go on a weight-loss journey for three months just so this guy could reevaluate things. Ha!

Audre is a gorgeous Black woman with a powerful presence. She's passionate about CrossFit and strength training, and she has a tall, curvy physique. What's ironic is that health is a value for her, too. She has a spunky personality and fire in her eyes. She uses her energy well, fighting for her clients and advocating for them in her role as a social worker.

If you took one look at Audre, you'd think people's comments about her body would just bounce off her, no problem. But Audre struggled with disordered eating habits in high school, and her boyfriend's rejection triggered old patterns for her.

When we started our work together, the first thing we did was go through her Negativity Loop. It looked like this:

- **Stressor:** her body shape
- **Thought:** *I can't change my body shape, no matter how hard I try.*
- **Emotion:** shame
- **Protection:** emotional eating and compensating at the gym

As Audre and I dug into the origin of her shame, she found the culprit. In high school, her friends bonded over diets and weight-loss

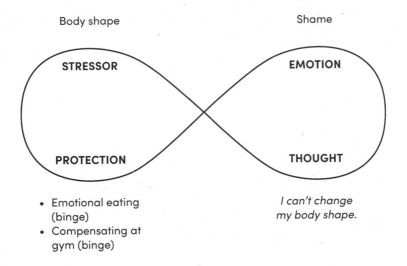

Body shape

Shame

STRESSOR

EMOTION

PROTECTION

THOUGHT

- Emotional eating (binge)
- Compensating at gym (binge)

I can't change my body shape.

solutions. (How sad is that?) At the time, this confused her. She'd never hated her body or wanted to change it. Her family was filled with strong matriarchs who all owned their figures. She read magazines that featured Black bodies of all shapes and sizes on the cover, celebrating excellence and accomplishment, not the ones she saw in grocery store lines that glorified thinness and featured the latest weight-loss fad.

In her house, food was family. Saying no to an extra helping would make her grandmother shake her head with a "tsk!" Southern comfort food was exactly that—*comforting*. The idea of restricting food in order to change her body was a culture shock to her.

Yet as she got older and experienced the racism wrapped up in diet culture,[8] she tried the diets and the exercise programs as a way of bonding with her friends. But as her friends got thinner, nothing changed for her. To feel better, she worked harder at the gym, and she staved off her shame with emotional eating.

When Audre first came to see me, we grieved the story of her feeling her body wasn't good enough. She had navigated much of her life feeling as though she wasn't thin enough or pretty enough, and not good enough overall. She needed space to process those feelings.

From there, Audre and I worked on interrupting her patterns. She was trying to escape her shame by turning to food—an avoidance protection response. The way to break that cycle was through attentiveness. Whenever she felt tempted to respond to negative feelings with emotional eating or going hard at the gym, she paused and asked herself, *What do I actually need from food? What do I need at the gym?* These questions helped her take charge instead of reacting.

When we started addressing Audre's false scripts, things began to change. She learned to see her body as a gift. She wanted to be like the strong matriarchs in her family, who went through hardship and survived, thanks to their strength. She embraced the idea of body inclusivity, which celebrates all body shapes, sizes, and abilities. Body positivity and inclusivity became her Joyful Purpose.

Audre protected her purpose within her social groups with a simple internal boundary. Any time her friends talked about weight loss or achieving a certain standard for beauty, she said internally, *Good for them, not for me.* And if she wanted to enjoy a brownie, she called out her Judge's voice and let herself eat a serving. She was able to enjoy foods she loved with her family and friends rather than eating in secret or bingeing on the entire plate until she felt sick.

Over the next several months, Audre learned to celebrate the differences in all bodies, including her own. And this celebration lit her up with defiant joy.

The next step was to make exercise a joyful experience. In her mind, the only exercise that counted involved intense workouts geared for weight loss. But this perspective was actually sabotaging her.

Michelle Segar, director of the University of Michigan's Sport, Health, and Activity Research and Policy Center, wanted to find out what kept people from being motivated to exercise. As part of a study, she asked forty women what made them feel happy and successful. Their answers were remarkably similar: to have meaningful connections, to feel relaxed, and to make progress on the goals they'd set for themselves. But one surprising finding emerged from her study. The women who were regular exercisers viewed exercise as something that helped them accomplish these desires. The women who didn't exercise viewed it as working *against* their desires. Segar reported that the women who had a narrow definition of exercise engaged in less movement.[9] In other words, when we view exercise merely as a vehicle to lose weight, we actually move our bodies *less.*

Audre was accustomed to moving her body as a means to change her body. She didn't move for the joy of it. After making a W.I.L.L., we identified an activity that helped her move her body and felt fun: dancing.

Now Audre takes dance classes instead of only doing high-impact fitness classes. Now that she's enjoying moving her body, she's taking better care of it.

When she came into my office to talk about this guy's text, we took time to grieve the breakup, and then we celebrated. We celebrated that his comments didn't derail her. Instead, she could recognize that his words were more about his own journey and had nothing to do with her. She was confident in who she was, and she had more important things to do than get pulled back into the life-sucking patterns of yo-yo dieting. She was living out her Joyful Purpose.

HOW TO LOVE YOUR BODY

Years ago, I (Carly) was fed up with not being able to lose weight. Desperate for a solution, I went to Google and typed, "how to love your body to lose weight." It's funny how in that fateful Google search, I was still focused on losing weight. I was tired of hating my body, but I didn't want to let go of the dream of weight loss.

But that search opened my eyes to a new way of looking at food, exercise, and my body. As I confronted my false scripts, I realized that whenever I tried to shrink myself, someone somewhere was making money off my shame. I remember thinking, *How much does it cost, in a dollar amount, for me to hate my belly fat that much? And who gets that money?* Every time I looked at my body in the mirror and wished it were different or "less," I thought less of myself.

Over time, I learned that I could love my body without losing weight and that doing so opened me up to more of the joy God had for me. Through nutritional counseling and my own work, I am learning to live out my Joyful Purpose with my body.

If you struggle to find freedom and joy when it comes to your body, here are some ways you can reframe the way you feel about it:

- Be more mindful about what's happening emotionally when it comes to your body and food. Instead of reacting to your emotions, pause. *(Be curious with your emotions.)*
- Discover how to correctly identify hunger cues and attune to the needs of your body. Instead of using an avoidance protection response, pay attention. *(Interrupt the loop.)*
- Commit to speaking kindly about your body and the way it moves you through the world. Start learning how to be your body's friend so you can keep it healthy and love it well. *(Call out the Judge.)*
- Vow to never self-harm again. No going on a strict diet, restricting food, and talking cruelly about the curves and lines on your sweet body. *(Interrupt the loop.)*
- Become discerning about the lies of diet culture. *(Challenge false scripts.)*
- See nutritious eating as a fun and enjoyable experience. *(Make it fun.)*

I don't consider my work in this area to be done. I'm still learning what it looks like to live out my own Joyful Purpose when it comes to my body and to empower our clients to experience this freedom too.

You might be thinking, *What if I'm doing keto, Whole30, WW [or any other weight-loss or wellness program]? Can I still do it with a Joyful*

Purpose? The answer is yes! *And* pay attention to your motivation behind the program. If you evaluate what's driving you and still feel these are working for you, then go for it. When you're triggered, or when you notice diet culture popping up in your story, identify your Negativity Loops and figure out what cycles need to be broken. If you determine that these programs are feeding into self-sabotaging patterns, pay attention. It's not about a simple *should* or *shouldn't*—that's for you to decide.

You may also be wondering if there are some people who actually *do* need a program. Yes, some people do. If you're in recovery from an eating disorder, then your relationship to food may be similar to having a broken bone that needs a cast. You need the structure and design of the cast until your bone sets and is completely healed. Once you're healed, you may need physical therapy to strengthen the muscles. When you no longer need a cast and you graduate from physical therapy, it's up to you to listen to your body and not push too hard. The same is true when it comes to a disordered relationship with food. Sometimes you need a guide, whether that's a nutritional counselor, a therapist, a therapy group, or a program, to help you heal your relationship with food when attunement with your body has been eroded.

It's possible to put the start-from-joy principles into practice and heal your relationship with food, exercise, and your body. When you heal the emotional patterns born from your story, you emerge on the other side resilient and confident. You can recognize that your body is a gift and that it's a privilege to take care of it.

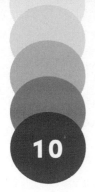

10 ENJOY YOUR MONEY

End the taboo surrounding money. Make a plan,
spend with confidence, and feel safe around money.

Kim was afraid—*terrified*, in fact. She was frozen at the kitchen island, palms sweating, head spinning. A small voice in her head was telling her she shouldn't be scared—she should trust that it would all work out. But her anxiety was louder than her confidence. *Will we be okay this month?* she wondered.

Meanwhile, her husband, Stephen, had a bounce in his step. He'd finally bought the patio furniture they'd been talking about. He couldn't wait to share his excitement with his wife.

Unfortunately, that's not what happened.

Kim attacked Stephen for recklessly spending money when they had a mortgage, bills, groceries, and other expenses. Stephen was furious that no matter how hard he worked, it never seemed like they had enough money for Kim.

"I make a lot of money," Stephen said. "I should feel free to spend it however I want to. I deserve it."

"But you spend without thinking about our family and what we actually need," Kim countered. "I wish you'd be more careful."

Kim and Stephen had different approaches to money. Kim was constantly worried about their finances. She wanted to save as much as possible, both for their goals and for any curveballs that might surprise them. Stephen, on the other hand, wanted to enjoy the fruits of his labor. He knew he made enough money—he just didn't want to think about it or talk about it.

Kim and Stephen both had an unhealthy relationship with money. They needed to ditch the emotional charge of this topic so they could pursue a bigger purpose together.

YOUR RELATIONSHIP WITH MONEY

Think about your money habits for a moment.

- When was the last time you checked your bank account?
- How much debt do you have?
- How much do you have in savings?
- When you hear the word *budget*, what feelings come up for you?
- When you think about money, what is your emotional response? Shame? Guilt? Fear?

Many of us have an unhealthy emotional relationship with money, and we often don't even realize it. When people go to see Carly, they talk about stressors such as arguing with a partner about finances, experiencing work stress, being afraid they won't be able to make ends meet, feeling taken advantage of or burned out in their jobs, or dealing with family members who ask for money. When she asks how their financial choices play a role, people are often surprised.

"Why would you ask that?" they ask. "That's super personal!"

Talking about money is almost as taboo as talking about sex and intimacy. But our false scripts around money are part of the undercurrent of so many life stressors. These false scripts, when left unchecked, result in unhealthy emotional relationships with money.

Here are some signs of an unhealthy relationship with money, along with the dimension of healthy living they impair:

- Your value is tied to your net worth. *(self-esteem)*
- You struggle to ask for help handling money; it's uncomfortable to talk about. *(self-care)*
- You overshare information about your financial situation. *(self-protection)*
- You never stray outside your budget and rarely give to causes that matter to you. *(self-protection)*
- You don't keep a budget because you avoid thinking about money. *(self-awareness)*
- You regularly get in fights with your partner about money. *(self-care)*
- You struggle with overspending or underspending. *(self-control)*
- You believe being a good person means rejecting the role of money in your life. *(self-esteem)*
- You refuse to let anybody pay for you, or you struggle to receive gifts. *(self-protection)*
- You love to splurge on other people, to your own detriment. *(self-control)*
- You think you shouldn't make a certain salary because you're not worth it. *(self-esteem)*
- You believe accepting more money for your passion is selling out. *(self-esteem)*
- You'd rather spend money to communicate love than connect emotionally. *(self-protection)*
- You feel stupid when talking about money. *(self-esteem)*
- You shrug off basic money matters as "adulting." *(self-esteem)*

- You overly rely on your partner or your family members to take care of money for you. *(self-care)*
- You can't prioritize when it comes to finances. Everything in your life, from bills to entertainment, has the same value assigned to it. *(self-awareness)*
- You have a separate bank account from your spouse because you're ashamed of your financial situation. *(self-care)*
- You hide what you buy from your family. *(self-protection)*

Actions like these, which are born from false scripts about money, damage our relationships and disempower us from taking care of ourselves. But money doesn't have to induce shame, guilt, or fear. You can break your unhealthy emotional patterns around money and create a new story around your finances.

A new story about money might look like this:

- finally getting out of debt
- being a team with your partner when it comes to money instead of constantly fighting about it
- saving money and investing in your future
- spending money in a way that matches your values and long-term goals
- expecting a fair salary for the work you do

Consider this: your greatest financial barrier might not be the amount of money you have but your *relationship* with money. This is a solvable problem, which means there's hope in this area of your life. Let's start by calling out the common false scripts around money.

FALSE MONEY SCRIPTS

I (Carly) admit that I don't have the best relationship with money. When I was in college and grad school, I didn't understand the scope of all the money I was pulling out in the form of loans, nor was I prepared to pay it off once Neal and I were in the real world. I just echoed the sentiments of my parents and the generations before me: "One day, you'll make enough to pay it off. Don't worry." So I kept pushing off all money talk into the future. I didn't want to think about finances while I was getting a degree to help people. *After all, I'm not doing it for the money*, I told myself. All this just perpetuated my ignorance about money.

I find that people in helping occupations often share a similar mindset about money: since we care about people, we shouldn't care about financial concerns. But I learned the hard way that you can assign as much moral value to ignorance about money as you want, but it still leads to destructive outcomes.

Jesus said, "No one can serve two masters. . . . You cannot serve both God and money."[1] Sometimes this verse is used to justify ignorance about financial wellness. We think that if we invalidate the role of money in our lives, we're serving a noble purpose. But when ignoring our finances leads us to not take care of ourselves or those we love, we *are* serving money. Financial stress plays in the background of our minds, guiding us to self-sabotage even when we don't realize it. The financial anxiety is always with us, living rent free.

Serving the master of money doesn't just mean loving wealth. It can mean ignoring financial wellness so much that it ends up controlling you and distracting you from your Joyful Purpose.

I knew I had to change my relationship with money. I had a big dream to build a large group-therapy practice, which would require wise financial stewardship. I wanted to be debt free. I wanted to give to causes that mattered to me. And I didn't just want to depend on Neal to handle our money; I wanted us to be a team.

I began exploring financial psychology and landed on the work of Drs. Brad and Ted Klontz, both of whom are considered pioneers in their field. In their book *Mind over Money*, they outline common money scripts that sabotage people. Money scripts are false beliefs you have about money and what will bring you happiness.[2] They come from our family, our friends, our culture, and past trauma. This book offers different names for money scripts, but in our work at Enjoyco, we call the two most common ones a money-mind script and a money-blind script. These are the saboteurs to watch out for in your relationship with money.

Money-Mind Script

I (Neal) grew up in a family where money was exalted as the savior for hard times. If only we could gain a large sum of money through the lottery or rigorous labor, we would be free of our difficult circumstances. This was my false script: *If we had more money, we'd be happy.* Or, put another way: *If we didn't have to worry about money, life would be great.*

We call this the money-mind script—where money is constantly on someone's mind. In this relationship with money, *having it* is the answer. People with a money-mind script tend to:

- think about money all the time, believing that having more is the solution to their problems
- experience anxiety about not having enough money
- spend money to feel connected to others
- feel like they need to have beautiful things as an expression of their identity
- spend more than they have by accident or just because "it's worth it"
- pursue career success (sometimes at the expense of everything else) because they believe their worth is tied to the money they make
- enjoy the thrill of shopping and spending
- believe that money will save their family
- spend money to help others feel more comfortable, to their own detriment

A money-mind script overemphasizes the role of money in your life. On a Negativity Loop, it would look something like this: you try to escape negative feelings by spending money, giving money, or working to make more money. People with a money-mind script pursue safety, security, love, and belonging through money. In doing so, they create an unhealthy emotional relationship with it.

A money-mind script has some benefits, when it's kept in check. People who hold on to this script typically think about money because they want to take care of the people in their lives. They want to solve other people's discomfort and help them feel safe, secure, and loved. These are qualities that should be celebrated. The trouble comes when people pursue the money-mind script to their own detriment. They work too much in an attempt to make more money, they spend money they don't have, or they spiral into anxiety over not having enough to take care of themselves and others. Along the way, money ends up consuming their minds.

God knows that worshiping money leads us to trust the wrong source for our joy, safety, security, and salvation. When the Hebrew people left Egypt after being slaves, they took their gold with them. In their impatience and anxiety for Moses to come down from Mount Sinai, they fashioned their gold into a calf statue. Then they worshiped it—they literally worshiped their money.[3]

It's easy to read this story and think, *I would never do something like that!* But we act similarly in our own lives. In our anxiety and impatience, we overwork. We stockpile our cash. We spend more just to feel better. To feel safe and secure, we elevate money to a role it was never supposed to have.

People who struggle with a money-mind script can benefit from examining their values to discern why they're spending money, working long hours, and feeling anxious about finances. When we see having more money as the answer to our happiness, the bar for our joy keeps moving further away. It may start with, "If only I made $3,000 more," and then it becomes $5,000 more, then $10,000 more, and so on. When we deny ourselves contentment with our money, it gets free reign to rule our minds.

Money-Blind Script

Just as rampant as the money-mind script—but more under the radar—is the money-blind script. This script goes like this: *If I avoid money, then I'll be happy.* People who have a money-blind script tend to:

- believe money (rather than the *love* of money[4]) is the root of all kinds of evil
- justify that they don't do things for the money
- believe money will corrupt them if they have too much
- avoid conversations about money
- joke with their friends about how poor they are
- feel uncomfortable about spending money on themselves
- save all their money
- avoid setting a budget

People with a money-blind script don't want to look at, think about, or engage with money at all. They might squirrel their money away so they don't have to look at it, or they might avoid basic actions of financial self-care such as setting a budget, investing, or checking their bank account.

As with a money-mind script, a money-blind script is not all bad. People with this script are masters at enjoying the present. They're not worried about not having enough. Not having money, in their minds, means they're good. They feel free to be generous with their time and talents, and they're willing to give themselves to causes that matter to them. This works to their disadvantage, however, when their lack of financial awareness leads them to neglect their needs.

The challenge for those with a money-blind script is to stay present with their money long enough to make wise decisions. This doesn't mean they have to become experts at all financial tasks. Those with this script usually do well when they automate their savings, bills, and investments so they can spend less time looking at their money while still having their needs met. Those with money-blind scripts also do well to seek counsel for managing their money.

Attentiveness is the solution to avoidance protection responses—the way to curb the detrimental effects of a money-blind script.

HOW TO GET HEALTHY WITH MONEY

So how can we break these patterns and learn to enjoy our finances in a healthy way? How can we break the emotional power of money and instead use it to take care of our needs and make the world a better place?

Violetta came to meet with me (Carly) because she was overwhelmed by financial stressors. In Violetta's mind, more money would solve her problems. Her strained relationship with her daughter, her mother's dependency, and her feelings of anxiety would all be solved if more money came rushing in like a waterfall.

Violetta was the single mother to her beautiful daughter, and she was the devoted daughter to her recently divorced mother. Her mother had never worked or brought home an income. Both Violetta and her mother benefited from the wealth of Violetta's dad and grandfather. But when her grandfather passed away and her dad abandoned their family, she was left to provide for her mother and her daughter on her own—something she was willing to do even though she was strapped for cash herself.

For years Violetta took care of her mother and her daughter, but the responsibility was starting to take a toll on her. Because her mother didn't feel empowered with money, she depended on Violetta for everything. Eventually, it became too much for Violetta to keep up with. Violetta kept pulling out her credit card to meet her mother's demands, and now she was in debt. Her mother's financial dependence was sabotaging the entire family. Violetta had to do something.

Violetta's Negativity Loop went like this:

- **Stressor:** not having enough money
- **Thought:** *I can't support everyone.*
- **Emotions:** guilt and shame
- **Protection:** overspending

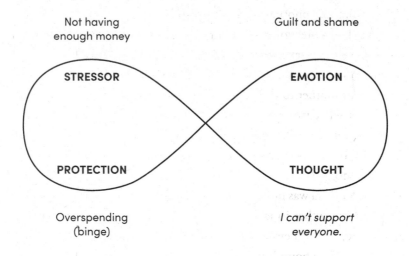

Not having enough money

Guilt and shame

STRESSOR   EMOTION

PROTECTION   THOUGHT

Overspending (binge)

I can't support everyone.

Violetta had a money-mind script. She thought having more money would mean her daughter and her mother would feel safe and secure. But if this pattern continued, Violetta would keep spending money she didn't have and feel unable to meet everyone's needs.

As I dug into the story behind her emotions, something stood out to me. When Violetta was growing up, she was quick to spend her money because if she saved it, her father would take it away. He used money as a carrot for good behavior, dangling it in front of her so she would behave and taking it away if she misbehaved. This approach to money backfired, because it only taught Violetta that money wouldn't stay. She learned a "use it or lose it" response—she had to spend her money the moment she got it, or it would be gone.

When Violetta became an adult, she immediately spent her money on her daughter and her mother. She loved the rush of spending, especially if it meant communicating love to her family.

Being generous to her family wasn't inherently the problem; in fact, that can be a good quality. What needed to be solved was Violetta's feeling that she never had enough for the things that actually mattered to her. Because she believed more money would solve her problems, there was always another tier to strive for.

Since her protection response was bingeing, we constructed boundaries to help her save money and take care of her daughter and her mother. Violetta still wanted to help her mother; she just didn't want to help her mother to the point that it hurt both of them.

Here's what we came up with: any time her mother asked for money, Violetta would communicate the boundary with something like this: "I can't give you money, but I can clean your house" or "I can't give you money, but I can help you look for a job." The genius of this was that Violetta was protecting herself and her family, but she was also helping her mother in the process. By not giving her mother money every time, Violetta empowered her to seek ways to make money herself. This simple boundary helped everyone.

We also made goals around spending when it came to Violetta's daughter. Instead of blindly pursuing more money, Violetta identified specific goals for her spending. In other words, she was learning to spend on purpose. She came up with fun activities such as going on a hot-air balloon ride with her daughter, and she saved money for those specific events.

Violetta's Joyful Purpose was to show her daughter that money didn't control her; rather, she had control over her money. The last thing she wanted her daughter to believe was that money could solve all problems and that if she blindly threw more money at a situation, everyone would be happy. She wanted to educate her daughter about finances so she wouldn't repeat the same patterns.

Violetta no longer feels like a bad mother and daughter. She's able to save for fun activities with her daughter, and because she has goals attached to her savings, she feels like she has enough to be the mother she wants to be. And in the process of setting boundaries with her mother, her mother was able to get a job.

Kim and Stephen (the couple at the beginning of the chapter who had opposite approaches to money) had a different challenge regarding finances.

While Kim had a money-mind script, Stephen had a money-blind script. They both needed to challenge their false scripts and trace how their stories had contributed. Kim grew up in a free-spirited family that didn't talk much about money, and Stephen grew up in a family that could never enjoy their money. They both were rebelling from the patterns they grew up with, and it resulted in new patterns that were sabotaging them.

After recognizing their false scripts, they had to interrupt their patterns. Kim's response led her to overthink money matters. She needed to place boundaries around when she would focus on money so it didn't remain an ongoing stressor in the background. Stephen had an avoidance protection response that led him to avoid looking at the budget. To help their family and align on their priorities, Stephen also needed to set aside time to think about money.

Their solution was to have a money meeting on the last Friday of every month. They now take time to review their expenses from the previous month, and then they set the budget for the next month. If at any point during the meeting they get emotionally triggered, they rely on the start-from-joy principle about being curious with their emotions. They take a moment to regulate themselves and then reengage with the conversation.

Now Kim and Stephen can enjoy money together—it doesn't hold power over them. Instead, it's a tool they use to build a life that's in alignment with their family's values.

HOW TO DEAL WITH CONFLICTING SCRIPTS

When Carly and I first got married, we spent two years in ignorant bliss about our finances. We were broke seminary students, and I worked hard to make the minimum payments on our debts. We weren't making much and we had a lot of school debt, but I was optimistic about our finances—I knew a promising future was ahead of us. I was growing my business, and soon Carly would be a licensed therapist. Life was looking bright.

But two years into our marriage, we got a message about an unpaid student debt Carly had. I was puzzled because I thought we had all her debt covered. When we logged into the account, my eyes grew big. I watched with horror as the amount of our total debt doubled before my eyes.

Carly was filled with shame. She didn't realize how much she'd been pulling out in student loans, and she didn't even know this loan existed. She burst into tears. Meanwhile, I was still pulling my jaw off the ground.

This was our financial "come to Jesus" moment. I knew things had to change. We would no longer continue in ignorance; it was time to get our financial life in order.

To accomplish this, however, we had to heal our relationship with money—both as individuals and as a couple. While Carly had a money-blind script, I had a money-mind script. This led me to work hard for money and shut Carly out of the financial picture. We were not a team.

Here are some steps we took to heal our relationship with money. If you are struggling in this area, they may be beneficial for you, too.

- **Learn how you approach money.** This involves diving into your Negativity Loops and understanding the false scripts that come into play for you. *(Challenge false scripts.)*

- **Create and follow a spending plan.** A budget might sound boring and restrictive to you. And we know that whenever we feel restricted from something, we end up overdoing it (the forbidden fruit syndrome). So consider creating a spending plan, which puts limits on your spending while also giving you enough freedom to not feel confined. *(Interrupt your loops.)*
- **Normalize money through routine conversations.** Money avoiders prefer to keep money a taboo topic. Yet the more it remains a secret, the more our shame, guilt, and fear increase. As Brené Brown says, "Shame loves secrecy."[5] Normalizing money means acknowledging there's nothing inherently shameful or wrong about money. We can talk about it, stay present with it, and treat it as a neutral part of life, not as something evil or negative. *(Call out the Judge.)*
- **Use soft, not harsh, start-ups.** If you and your partner have conflicting Negativity Loops, be intentional about using soft start-ups for your conversations around money. A study by relationship experts John Gottman and Sybil Carrère found that conversations tend to end on the same note they begin on.[6] Rather than beginning a conversation with a harsh start-up ("I can't believe you did that!"), practice a soft start-up such as, "Hey, can I check something out with you?" Opening money conversations in gentle ways helps ensure a productive conversation. *(Interrupt your loops; be curious with emotions.)*
- **Pay for what you value.** Spending money on things that fit your values doesn't just mean giving to causes you care about. Studies suggest that spending money on experiences makes us happy.[7] Other studies say that spending money on things that save time also makes us happy.[8] *(Make it fun.)*

Years after the student-loan revelation, we paid off most of our debt, scaled our income, bought our dream house, and built a business. We're now able to consistently give to the causes that matter to us. And it all started with changing our relationship to money.

Our culture tells us that money should be worshiped or feared. On one extreme is the view that money is the end goal of every life—if you gather more of it, you'll finally have everything you want. On the other extreme, it's seen as a necessary evil of adulthood, and we can bond with others by connecting over our financial inadequacy.

Neither view of money is accurate. Money is just money. When we heal our financial relationship and put money in its proper place, we can use it to create the life we want.

It's not about having more money or less money. It's about relating to it differently. That means our financial circumstances don't determine our joy. We do.

It's not about having

more money or less money.

It's about relating

to it differently.

11 ENJOY YOUR WORK

Stop the pain with work. Explore your calling,
love what you do, and reinvent the 9-to-5.

During my time in therapy, I (Neal) made a drastic—some might say bizarre—decision.

My chief accountant was stunned by the news. "You did *what?*"

"I dissolved my business," I repeated with so much certainty that several people in the coffee shop turned their heads.

"But . . . why? The business was doing amazing."

I reached for my cup and quieted my voice. "Because it was time for me to stop overidentifying with my success. I don't want my self-worth to ride the highs and lows of my business. I just don't want to do this anymore."

My accountant had good reason to be shocked. It was a hasty decision. I also told him I'd accepted a new job doing work that seemed like a backward step in my career. It didn't make sense. But people like me with binge protection responses often respond to stress with extreme actions. The only step that made sense to me was to get out of my business as fast as possible. I thought a move like this would heal my relationship with work.

Then, shortly after I started my new job, my friend Blake and I grabbed lunch at a local pho restaurant. As I shoveled noodles into my mouth, I expressed my discontentment about my new job.

"This new position just isn't satisfying me," I told Blake. "It has all the makings of a lifelong career, but it doesn't light me up like my business did."

Everyone deserves a friend like Blake—one who listens enough to read between the lines and offer a challenging perspective. Blake ate his pho at a slow pace, as if he were trying to digest my words in addition to what was in his bowl. After several minutes of listening to my dissatisfaction, he stopped me.

"It sounds like you're unhappy because this isn't where you thought you would be in your life now. But what stops you from being happy *here*?" This question was followed by another slurp of noodles.

"What do you mean?" I was confused, because I thought I'd just explained what would make me happy.

Blake was smart enough to know that the things I was talking about were just symptoms of something deeper. "Neal. I've been in your life through a lot of transitions now. You approach work the same way," he said. "You look to your work to provide your worth. This job title isn't what you expected for yourself, and that's valid, but that means nothing for your worth. Work isn't everything."

My noodles slipped through my chopsticks at Blake's mic-drop statement. "Explain more," I said.

"Your work isn't meant to fully satisfy you. The more you believe it will, the more discontentment you'll feel at your job. Lean into this season. It's clear you're here for a reason. Maybe it's just to let go of past work patterns or to find healing in other areas. Regardless, I think you need to take this opportunity to find value in other parts of your life."

I felt Blake's words rattle me to my bones.

After that transformational lunch, I stopped looking for a quick escape from my job. Instead, I committed myself to rediscovering other parts of my life—the parts that had been lost when I made my business everything.

It was a hard lesson, but I eventually learned that I'm worthy outside my professional success. I wouldn't have arrived at this revelation if I hadn't explored my relationship with work.

• • •

In 2019, Anthony Klotz, an associate professor of management at Texas A&M, predicted that a "great resignation" was coming. What no one knew at the time was that a global pandemic was on the verge of redefining work everywhere. Now the great resignation is here. Between April and June of 2021, a total of 11.5 million workers quit their jobs. And this trend doesn't seem to be slowing down.[1]

Citing reasons such as burnout, a toxic work culture, and fears about cost cutting, millions of employees have been rethinking what they want from their work. And many people didn't have the luxury of asking these questions—their work status changed because they were furloughed or fired and left without jobs.

Now millions of people are evaluating their priorities when it comes to work and their physical, emotional, and family health. Employers are desperately trying to find ways to combat increased turnover, while employees are asking themselves hard questions about their jobs: *What's really necessary? And what do I want?*

Maybe you, too, have been doing some reevaluating when it comes to your job. There has never been a better time to explore your relationship with work and build a work situation—whether at your current job or at a new job—that fits your values.

When you heal your relationship with work, you can:

- go to work without being afraid of the day ahead
- create healthy boundaries that have you ending work on time
- feel confident and courageous enough to ask for what you need at work
- align your values with your work
- stay engaged at your job and find greater enjoyment in your weekly routine

If you've been feeling discouraged or weary when it comes to work, we want you to know there's another way. It all starts with healing your relationship with work.

REDEFINING WORK

The following signs indicate an unhealthy emotional relationship with work, along with the dimension of healthy living they impair:

- You stay in an unhealthy work environment longer than you should. *(self-protection)*
- You struggle to unplug during off hours. *(self-protection)*
- You constantly switch jobs in search of the perfect one. *(self-control)*
- You don't know what you want or like in a job. *(self-awareness)*
- Your value is wrapped up in your job title. *(self-esteem)*
- You don't ask for what you need to be successful in your job. *(self-care)*
- You feel like you don't have what it takes to do a new job, so you stay stuck where you are. *(self-awareness)*
- You feel like you're following a script when it comes to your job instead of doing what you want to do. *(self-awareness)*

- You constantly feel resentful toward your boss, your coworkers, or your peers. *(self-care; self-protection)*
- You work long hours even when there isn't a pressing deadline. *(self-control)*
- You're not generous with your time at work. You show up, do the bare minimum, and leave. *(self-protection)*
- You rarely take vacations from your work. *(self-protection)*

By now you know what causes an unhealthy relationship in this area of your life. That's right—false scripts.

Imagine work on a spectrum. On the left side are those who view work as a means to an end. There's no significance other than getting a paycheck so they can enjoy life outside their job. "Work hard to play hard" might be their mantra. On the right side are those who view work as giving their lives ultimate meaning. Since work provides them with a sense of identity and worth, they pour every bit of their lives into their career. They can't wait for someone to ask, "So, what do you do?"

I (Carly) lived on the left side of this spectrum. My script had always been "Work is hard." I just wanted to show up, do the parts I loved, and then go home. If an assignment was too tedious or made me feel a difficult emotion, I would procrastinate, avoid it, or grin and bear it until I could do something more fun.

Neal, on the other hand, lived on the right side of this spectrum. He loved a challenge at work. And when he wasn't working, he was involved with a passion project on the side. I came home never wanting to talk about, think about, or acknowledge work. I hid my work-avoidance tendency under the guise of "relaxing." Neal, meanwhile, was excited to talk about the new ideas and strategies he was thinking about.

This made for some interesting Negativity Loops at our dinner table: I avoided work, while he loved work too much. Neither end of the spectrum is healthy; they're both the result of false scripts.

After helping dozens of clients sort through their beliefs about work, we've identified two of the most common false scripts that relate to work:

- **Work Evader:** The work evader thinks, *I'll be happy when I don't have to work.* There isn't much purpose, passion, or enjoyment tied to their job. It's something they have to get through. They are often insecure at work, so they don't feel safe speaking up or taking risks.
- **Workaholic:** The workaholic thinks, *I'll be happy once I'm successful.* They look to work for their sense of safety and security, and they only feel like they have purpose when they're achieving their goals. They look to their success to provide their confidence and happiness.

Let's break down these two false scripts and see how they can wreak havoc on your work life.

Work Evader

If you're a work evader, you may struggle with an emotional relationship that leaves you saying, "How can I get out of this?" or "I'm just counting down the days to my next vacation." Sometimes it's not just that you don't want to work; it's that you don't feel confident in your ability to contribute at your job. It's easier to avoid trying too hard so you don't have to risk failing. With this script, we become victims of joyless work—enduring anxious days and dragging ourselves to the office Monday through Friday. This compounds our Negativity Loop, making every task seem harder than it is.

Over the course of a lifetime, we spend more than 90,000 hours working, which breaks down to one-third of our lives.[2] If we hold on to a work-evader script, it means forfeiting a large portion of our lives to unhappiness. There is no better picture of this false script than the modern notion of retirement. We're incentivized to work hard and save so that one day we'll no longer have to work. We can enjoy a lush, rich life doing whatever we want . . . but only after work ends.

Retirement isn't bad by any means. For most people, it's a time of reaping the good seeds they've sown. But this view of delaying happiness until retirement is a by-product of how our culture at large views work. The emphasis is on life outside our jobs, and the payoff is getting more time to spend outside of work. The false script of "I will be happy when I no longer have to work" means we avoid finding joy in the here and now. It robs us of feeling confident, hopeful, and purposeful about what we can contribute to the world with our skills and talents.

The work-evader script results in avoidance responses toward work, but it also leads to binge responses under the guise of relaxation and rest. Avoidance responses include not giving our best, not risking, not trying new things (which can deaden our sense of passion and fulfillment), hopping from job to job, and using external medicators such as alcohol and food to numb feelings. Binge responses include bingeing activities outside of work, such as watching Netflix. People who struggle with a binge response feel as though they lack rest from their job, so they seek control by bingeing on rest activities.

If this is your belief system, it's no wonder work is hard and lacks purpose and fun. When we bring our skills and passions into the workplace, we can better advocate for our needs at work and enjoy what we do.

Workaholic

While our society often promotes the work-evader script, it also proclaims a competing message: that we should give everything to our jobs. Workaholics struggle with an emotional relationship with work that leaves them saying, "My career equals my safety, my security, and my success" or "Who am I without my job?" With this script, we overidentify with work and what it says about us. This compounds our

Negativity Loop, making every promotion, task, or project seem more important than it really is.

This script often leads to bingeing and rage responses. The bingeing responses include overworking and overidentifying with work. Then there are the rage responses. When people see their work as more important than it is, they blame other people for failing to match their level of commitment or they make them scapegoats whenever there's a setback. They might have a pattern of blaming their team or their coworkers for mistakes at work instead of taking ownership. In some cases, workaholics job hop (an avoidance response) when their job doesn't fully satisfy them.

A recent survey found that almost half of Americans consider themselves to be workaholics.[3] It's not hard to understand why this is a common script. We see a philosophy of hustle and meritocracy everywhere. If you scroll through social media or flip on the television, you'll encounter stories of rags-to-riches entrepreneurs who sacrificed everything to achieve their success. We praise these individuals and turn them into role models, yet in many cases, they're not good examples of healthy living.

When we seek to control our circumstances, our security, or our image by overworking, we have to shrink the rest of our lives to make space for work. Things like family, church, friends, and hobbies get pushed out of the circle. Work fills every inch, and we miss the joy of experiencing success in multiple areas of life.

A recent study by the Yale Center for Emotional Intelligence found that 20 percent of workers reported being highly engaged in their jobs, but this came at the risk of burnout.[4] When we follow this script and give our all to work, we end up dissatisfied and exhausted.

JOY IN WORK; JOY IN REST

As I (Neal) think about humans' relationship with work, I'm reminded that in the Bible, God gave Adam and Eve the call to work. This wasn't part of the Curse; it was something God established in a perfect world.[5] What this means is that when approached in a healthy way, work can be deeply satisfying. I'm also reminded that even God rested on the seventh day of creation.[6] Taking a day off work each week gives us the opportunity to acknowledge our human limitations and put our sense of security in God.

From the beginning of the Bible, we're presented with the idea that we're called to contribute to the world through our work but also that we're called to rest from that work. There is joy in work *and* joy in rest. This allows us to have a healthy, balanced approach to what we do.

So how can we heal our relationship with work? How can we break our patterns of overwork or work avoidance? How can we learn to love the one-third of our lives we spend working?

The answer is not simply to find happiness by changing your circumstances. It's learning how you relate to work and then making wise decisions to interrupt unhealthy patterns.

WHEN TO LEAVE YOUR JOB

Jordan thought he'd secured his ideal job. Right out of college he got a job in ministry, doing work that aligned with his values and passions. He was living the dream . . . or so he thought.

As with any job, there were some responsibilities he didn't enjoy. Unfortunately, these parts made up the majority of his day. These tasks began to eat at the core of his being, draining his energy and depleting his passion. By the time he came to my (Carly's) office, he was seeking treatment for his growing anxiety and depression.

"I don't get it," he told me in his first session. "I'm in a constant fog. I feel overwhelmed even before I get out of bed. The thought of spending social energy I don't have drains me even more. At work, I get distracted and then feel stupid when I can't respond to emails in a timely manner. I can't seem to get my tasks completed. But this was my dream job, and I'm doing tasks I know I'm good at and studied for in college. Why do I feel this way? Should I quit?"

It was a heavy question. Maybe you've found yourself in a similar situation.

Jordan's Negativity Loop was easy to spot:

- **Stressor:** the stable job he's "supposed" to have
- **Thought:** *This is a good job. I should be happy.*
- **Emotion:** fear of risk and change
- **Protection:** staying in the job, but spinning in worry and depression; asking everyone else's opinion without considering his own dreams

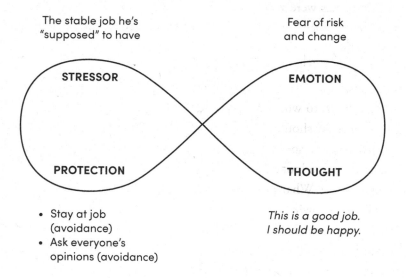

The stable job he's "supposed" to have

Fear of risk and change

STRESSOR

EMOTION

PROTECTION

THOUGHT

- Stay at job (avoidance)
- Ask everyone's opinions (avoidance)

This is a good job. I should be happy.

Jordan's protection responses were avoidance measures. He avoided his feelings of fear by staying in his job, even though it was slowly eating away at him. He asked his parents, peers, and mentors for their opinions, but this was just a way to avoid his inner world. He was tuned in to what everyone else wanted for his life without taking notice of his own heart.

As we dug into his story, we noted a pattern: Jordan's parents also stayed at jobs they hated for too long. He was dealing with some pesky lies that stirred guilt, shame, and fear:

- If you want to have a family one day, you need to find a steady job that will make a lot of money—and you won't be successful until you do.
- Work isn't supposed to be fun. That's why it's called *work*.
- Why take a risk when you have a good thing? Keep your head down and just do what you need to do.

These lies were working in the background of Jordan's mind any time he considered leaving his job. If he didn't explore his work scripts, he'd end up repeating his parents' pattern.

Jordan lacked self-awareness, and this was creating an unhealthy relationship with work. He needed to stop running from his inner reality and listen to what he wanted instead of following shaming voices about what he should be doing.

Jordan and I spent the majority of our time building self-awareness skills. First, we looked at the burnout in his current job. What was going wrong? What protections were sabotaging him? In what ways was he not showing up as his full self?

From there, we looked at what he *did* want in a job. He learned about his strengths and interests through tools like the Kolbe assessment and the StrengthsFinder test. We examined what other possible career paths he could explore and how they would align with a Joyful Purpose for his life. He learned practical strategies to ask for what he needed at work. And he built new boundaries so he could interrupt the false scripts that were sabotaging him, including the lie that he had to stay in this particular job to be safe and secure.

After several months of evaluating his strengths and his current work situation, Jordan took a risk and left his stable job. Soon after, he found a better job that allowed him to pursue his long-term dreams while also meeting his financial needs. He has rhythms of work and rest to keep burnout and depression at bay. And he built a W.I.L.L. that includes practices such as walking around outside during his lunch break, eating fueling foods in the morning, and starting each workday with the same enjoyable rhythm. He told me that this is the first time he's felt confident in a job, believing that what he does really makes a difference in his new company. He's building a life he loves—one that doesn't depend on what anyone else thinks.

Of course, you shouldn't leave a job just because it doesn't make you feel happy all the time. But when you're dealing with a chronic situation that is compromising your health, it might be time to consider a change. Before you make that leap, however, do the work of becoming self-aware. Ask yourself the hard questions that help tune you in to what you truly want for your life. This is how you can end burnout and build a work situation you enjoy.

WHEN TO STAY AT YOUR JOB

Veronica was facing a midlife crisis. She was fast approaching her fifties and she still hadn't found a job she loved. Instead, she was still job hopping. Her average tenure at a job was a year and a half—sometimes even shorter if another opportunity caught her eye. She wouldn't allow herself to be happy until she found a job that made the skies part and gave her constant butterflies. But this pattern never satisfied her the way she thought it would. She was constantly searching for meaningful work that would fulfill her.

In my (Carly's) time with Veronica, we talked about what she really wanted from her job.

"Happiness," she responded immediately.

What she didn't realize, however, was that she could find joy in the job she was currently in.

Her Negativity Loop looked like this:

- **Stressor:** boredom at work
- **Thought:** *Maybe this isn't the right place for me—there must be something better out there. I shouldn't have to settle.*
- **Emotions:** anger about still not knowing the best path for her life; fear of feeling stuck at her job; fear of missing out
- **Protection:** quitting and finding a new job

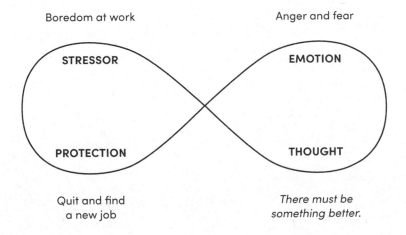

Boredom at work · Anger and fear · STRESSOR · EMOTION · PROTECTION · THOUGHT · Quit and find a new job · There must be something better.

Veronica had a workaholic script, even though she had a habit of job hopping. Her false script caused her to put too much value in her work, so when it didn't fully satisfy her, she left.

I (Neal) resonate with Veronica's pattern. In a culture that worships following your passion, it can be hard to stay at a job where your days are marked more by ordinary tasks than dramatic accomplishments.

Dr. Amy Wrzesniewski, professor at the Yale School of Management, made a critical discovery about the way people view their

**Wise actions
are often the result of slow,
well-thought-out decisions.**

work. According to her studies, we perceive our work in one of three ways:

- as a job that's good for pay and benefits—nothing more
- as a career for seeking advancement and success
- as a calling where we find meaning, purpose, and a sense of identity

Wrzesniewski and her team found that those who viewed their jobs as a calling were more engaged and found more personal satisfaction in their work. They reported that they would do their work even if they weren't paid.

For many people, the temptation is to find a job that immediately feels like a calling. But Wrzesniewski found something that contradicts this idea. She assumed passion would be the greatest predictor for seeing work as a calling. But in her study of college administrative assistants, she discovered that the assistants were not passionate about their jobs when they started. Instead, the primary predictor of a work-as-a-calling orientation was the number of years spent on the job. In other words, the longer they stayed and gained mastery in their discipline, the happier they were with their jobs. Passion follows mastery.[7]

Constantly searching for the job that will make you happy is an avoidance protection response. You might be trying to escape the shame of an unwanted identity, the fear of being unhappy, or the guilt of not being fulfilled at your job. But those feelings will inevitably follow you to a new job.

Now that's not to say we should never leave a job. But instead of jumping to the next shiny opportunity, we can benefit from creating a pause between our emotion and our protection response. We don't have to leave a job that isn't making us happy right away. Instead, we can bring attention to the parts of our job we want to avoid so we can deal with the emotions that urge us to make a change.

Wise actions are often the result of slow, well-thought-out decisions. If we can sit in the pause and truly understand the actions we're taking, then we can create more happiness and fulfillment in our professional lives.

Like Jordan, Veronica struggled with self-awareness. Because of childhood messages, she avoided her dream of going to fashion school. She wanted a job that felt like an instant calling, but she was just avoiding her real dream of doing fashion. In our work together, we dove into her passions and used what she loved about fashion to craft a Joyful Purpose. She found a job that checked enough of her boxes, and she's been able to stick with it while pursuing fashion in her free time.

WHEN WORK IS TOO MUCH

Ross was a vice president in his company—a place he had worked for fifteen years. He had three kids at home, and his wife was able to pursue her own interests and passions along with caring for the kids. He felt a lot of pride that he was able to financially provide for his family, but there was a problem. He was coping with the long hours, high expectations, and pressures of running a team of 150-plus employees by overworking and overdrinking. He hated to admit it, but he didn't know how to stop.

His Negativity Loop with work was intense:

- **Stressor:** pressure from higher-ups to meet year-end goals
- **Thought:** *It's all up to me—at work and at home.*
- **Emotion:** fear that the team won't make it and he'll take the blame; shame that he's not good enough for the job
- **Protection:** overworking; overdrinking; criticizing himself and his team

In addition to his binge protection response (overworking and overdrinking), Ross also had a rage protection response. When he fell

Pressure to meet
year-end goals

Fear and shame

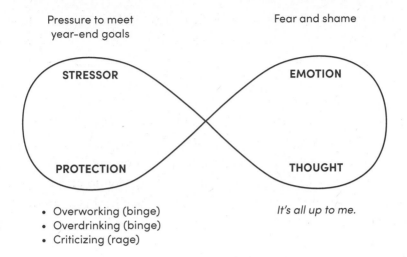

STRESSOR

EMOTION

PROTECTION

THOUGHT

- Overworking (binge)
- Overdrinking (binge)
- Criticizing (rage)

It's all up to me.

behind at work, he was overly critical of himself, thinking, *Get your act together!* He was raging against himself. But of course, this rage also spilled out into his relationships. His criticisms of his team made the work culture tense. And he brought his stress home, taking his anger out on his wife and kids. His life was spiraling out of control, and he had to do something.

Because Ross overidentified with his work, he couldn't bear the shame of not reaching his work goals. Not only that, but he feared that everything depended on him—both the company goals and the welfare of his family. The pressure was too much to bear, so he used alcohol to try to lighten it.

Now Ross is getting help with his alcoholism and workaholism in a recovery program at his church. To solve his binge responses, he's working with me (Carly) to set healthy limits in his work and his life. He's learning to acknowledge his emotions and meet them with compassion and care instead of criticism.

Ross's wife is going to therapy as well, exploring her own work messages so she can get a job now that her kids are going to college. She's tapping into parts of her that are waking up after a long time. This helps Ross feel supported so he can lighten up the pressure on himself. Now he and his wife are a team.

When work is too much, it's natural to dive into controlling measures. These actions don't have to be as intense as drinking, blaming, and criticizing; they could be as simple as procrastinating, working longer hours, or becoming overly rigid in your routines. Whatever your protection response might be, it's helpful to pay attention to these actions. Ask yourself what they're solving for you, and then take wise measures to interrupt them. This will bring you to a more joyful place when work is too much.

HOW TO HEAL YOUR WORK MESSAGES

Like Ross, I (Neal) overidentified with my work. Childhood wounds led me to double down on a fabricated image of success for myself, as if it proved my worth and significance in the world. Yet all I was doing was destroying my resilience at work. Because work was my identity, any setback in my professional life bruised my ego. Everything was too personal for me, all because I believed work was my life. It took several years, but I slowly healed my emotional relationship with work.

I learned a few key actions that might help you if you need to heal this relationship too:

- **Address the origins of your hard emotions.** Identify the unhelpful scripts you learned about work from your family or culture so you can find out what makes work difficult for you. *(Challenge false scripts.)*
- **Stop advertising your job title.** If you tend to overidentify with work, you may want to stop sharing what you do with other people for a while. This will help you put a pause between your emotions and your response. *(Interrupt your loops.)*
- **Take a social media break.** It's easy to highlight your successes and best moments on social media. Taking a break may help

you learn to be less of a "brand" and stay true to your real, authentic self. *(Interrupt your loops.)*

- **Identify your Joyful Purpose.** Here's my Joyful Purpose for work: "To become the rising tide that raises all ships." For too long, I believed I had to do things on my own to achieve success. But this belief put too much pressure on me to be successful at work. I realized that I didn't want to win alone; I wanted to share my success with others. As I pursued success and joy at work, others around me would become the best versions of themselves as well. *(Find your Joyful Purpose.)*

- **Say yes to jobs that align with your purpose.** By using your purpose as a filter for opportunities, you can recover your sense of joy and play when it comes to work. This means that you won't need work to prove your worth or help you reach the next marker of success. *(Make it fun.)*

As we pursue a healthy relationship with work, we need to remember that joy isn't a result of our circumstances; it's something God plants inside us. Our best work happens when we let our values, strengths, and passions inform the work we do. When we bring these values to the surface, we experience the alignment that makes a healthy work relationship possible.

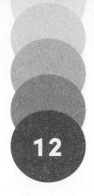

12 ENJOY YOUR RELATIONSHIPS

Let go of negative relationship patterns. Add greater love, intimacy, and joy to all your relationships.

"I'm *done.*"

I (Carly) watched as my client Chelsea sank into the couch, defeated. Her head leaned back as though weighed down by her thoughts. I adjusted myself in my chair, knowing I was about to engage some deep-seated beliefs. I was mentally rolling back my sleeves.

Chelsea had a pattern. Ever since her divorce, it seemed like she had a gravitational pull toward the wrong guys. In her search for "the one," she kept dating guys who were emotionally unavailable and who weren't interested in long-term relationships. As a result, her hopelessness about dating compounded.

I knew that dating in your forties isn't like dating in your twenties. It can be exhausting. But I also knew that Chelsea wasn't helping her case by going back to the same type of guys. Anytime she chose a guy who wasn't interested in a relationship, she confirmed her bias that dating was hard.

Chelsea had a fiery personality, flowing brown hair, and eyes that could slice you to pieces. She was also drop-dead gorgeous.

So why didn't she believe she was an absolute catch?

"Chelsea," I started, "do you know it's a *privilege* for guys to date you?"

"Then why am I in my forties and single?" she shot back.

She leaned forward and brought her hands to her face, massaging her temples as if she were fighting off a headache—or fighting off the lies that had taken root in her brain.

Chelsea struggled with a false script around relationships: that to be happy, she had to be married by age forty. When that didn't happen, her fears about being unworthy and unchosen took root.

Most people think finding joy is about changing your circumstances. But joy in relationships isn't about finding "the one," having sex, or having kids. It's about changing the way you view relationships so your deepest connections can yield hope, purpose, and delight.

As you do this work, your relationships will be marked by greater love, intimacy, and connection.

- You and your spouse will engage in more productive conflict that draws you closer together rather than farther apart.
- You'll be able to date from a place of confidence and freedom instead of fear as you search for a companion.
- Your children will be empowered to become strong, interdependent, and emotionally healthy adults.
- You will enjoy friendships that are vulnerable, trustworthy, and fun.

Relationships of all kinds are messy. They can be the source of some of our biggest stressors and disappointments—but they can also be our biggest sources of joy.

RELATIONSHIP CHECKUP

Have you ever stopped and asked yourself, *Why do my relationships bring me more stress than joy? Why do I keep repeating the same unhealthy relational patterns?*

Paying attention to your relationship to relationships can be difficult. But this is simply about seeing the way your relationships affect your emotional well-being. Healthy relationships are marked by interdependence with your loved ones—you can share yourself without losing yourself, and you can mutually depend on one another. Unhealthy relationships, on the other hand, can look like codependency, isolation, a lack of vulnerability, oversharing, or overidentifying.

Here are some signs of an unhealthy emotional relationship with relationships:

- You fear conflict, so you keep everything at surface level. *(self-protection)*
- You put your entire worth and value in your friendships, dating relationship, marriage, or children. *(self-esteem)*
- You struggle to trust anyone other than yourself. *(self-care; self-protection)*
- You rely too much on others to regulate your emotions and meet your needs. *(self-care)*
- You fear vulnerability and hide your emotions. *(self-protection)*
- You use relationships to cope with the stresses of life. *(self-control)*
- You don't experience sexual intimacy with your partner. *(self-protection)*
- You feel your child's emotions too deeply. *(self-protection)*
- You're quick to blame others instead of taking ownership in your relationships. *(self-awareness)*
- You overshare, vent, and complain about private matters of your life. *(self-protection)*

- You never have a preference when people ask where you want to go or what you want to do. *(self-awareness)*
- You keep dating emotionally unhealthy people. *(self-awareness)*
- You explode in anger at those closest to you. *(self-control)*
- You don't have any deep relationships. *(self-protection)*

If you see yourself in the list above, chances are that false scripts are to blame for your unhealthy relationships.

In our work with people who are struggling in their relationships, we've identified some of the most common false scripts:

- Being in a dating relationship will make you happy.
- Having your sexual needs met will make you happy.
- You don't need anyone else to be happy.
- All you need is your family to be happy.
- Raising your kids is the ultimate form of happiness.
- Once you're married, you'll live happily ever after.
- Being conflict free in your relationships equals happiness.

If we were to map these false scripts on a spectrum, on the left side would be scripts that say relationships are everything for happiness and success. If you buy into these scripts, you overidentify in your relationships. Overidentifying might mean relying on relationships to feel better about yourself or a situation. It also might mean engaging in people-pleasing or doing anything to keep the peace. The fear of being abandoned or disappointed results in a lack of boundaries and compromised self-care.

If you buy into the scripts on the right side of this spectrum, you undervalue the role of relationships. You exaggerate your independence and underidentify in your relationships. Underidentifying might mean not leaning on others when you need them and instead trying to take care of everything yourself. You may not believe other people can be trusted, especially if you've been hurt in the past. You may push people away or shut them down when they try to get too close.

When we swing to either extreme, relationships become our greatest stressors and disappointments. But there's a way to get back to the healthy middle—to a place where our relationships resonate with joy and flood our lives with happiness.

WHAT'S TRUE ABOUT RELATIONSHIPS

There are three foundational truths that confront the most common false scripts around relationships. Whether your false scripts lead you to stay guarded, put your hopes and dreams in others, or keep everything surface level, these truths will help you find a healthy balance in your relationships.

1. Relationships are worth the risk.

When I (Neal) was helping Robert share the results of his happiness study with the world, I was struck by the simplicity of his findings: that good relationships make us happier and healthier. We need people in our lives—not just work colleagues or immediate family, but an engaged community of people who really know us.

While many of us know this, we hit roadblocks along the way. Relational trauma, Western society's value of independence, and our own pride can lead us to reject help from others when we're in need. We feel apathetic about engaging in community, or we become convinced that having close relationships will only invite hurt and betrayal.

God created us with an innate desire to belong.[1] Research proves that our need for connection is a powerful motivation that's woven into the fabric of our being.[2] The more we lean into this intentional design, the happier and healthier we are.[3] Good relationships matter, and when you find the right people, they're worth the risk.

When we live outside this design, however, it's detrimental to our health and happiness. In an article in the *Harvard Business Review*,

Dr. Vivek H. Murthy, surgeon general of the United States, wrote, "Loneliness and weak social connections are associated with a reduction in lifespan similar to that caused by smoking 15 cigarettes a day and even greater than that associated with obesity."[4]

It's one thing to hear what studies say. But when you've been betrayed, hurt, abandoned, or shamed in relationships, none of this research matters. The only thing that seems clear is that the safest approach is to avoid investing too much in relationships. We self-protect by resisting attachments and not letting others into our lives.

There's a reason God gave us the desire to be in community with people. In her book *Love Sense*, Dr. Sue Johnson writes, "Emotional connection is a sign of mental health. It is emotional isolation that is the killer."[5] It's through emotional connection and healthy relationships that we cure loneliness, achieve happiness, and cultivate health.

2. Relationships can't fully satisfy you.

I (Carly) was meeting with a pregnant client who told me that she'd never felt truly loved before. She had so much love to give, and she wanted that unconditional love in return. In fact, the thing that excited her most about having a baby was finally having someone who would love her without fail.

As she spoke, I heard her longing for love so clearly. But I also knew she was looking for that love in the wrong place. Of course she would experience love in this new relationship. But she was placing this child on a pedestal, hoping they would fulfill all her needs. But a day will come when her baby learns the word *no* and screams, "I hate you, Mommy!" And one day that child will get to the teenage phase and eventually leave for college. No human being can bear the full weight of another person's emotional satisfaction.

When we talk about relationships, it's important to realize that not every need can be met by someone else. This is where Disney messed us up. We've been sold the fairy-tale scenario that all we need is a prince (or a princess) to solve our problems, and then we'll live happily ever after. But human relationships are built to disappoint.

Think about it: when God created human beings, he acknowledged, "It is not good for the man to be alone."[6] But he didn't just create a couple and stop there. He created each person to be in a relationship with him first and to glorify him.[7] As we image God, who is three in one, we reflect his relational nature—not just with one another, but with him.

God designed us to need a variety of relationships, calling us to love him first and then our neighbor as ourselves. We need to learn how to love all three: God, others, and the beautiful self he made. If we put unrealistic expectations on others, whether it's a spouse, a child, or a friend, we'll doom our relationships. We need to be proactive in building communities, support systems, and our own self-care habits so our needs can be met from multiple relationships instead of putting the burden on one individual.

My pregnant client had no close relationships outside her husband, which signaled to me that she would expect to have her needs met by a very narrow family unit, which was sure to let her down. If she had a support system of close friendships and deep emotional connection with God, herself, and others, then she could handle even the toughest ups and downs in her growing family. Part of her homework in therapy was to take intentional action to build a village around her, especially as she transitioned into this new role as a mother.

We need to bolster our relational tool belts so we can build a healthy tribe around us. It's through healthy relationships that we achieve all God has set out for us.

3. Failure is necessary; repair is everything.

In an attempt to keep the peace in our relationships, we might avoid conflict. We also might keep things shallow because we're afraid to dive into vulnerable territory. But all this does is create superficial relationships. Conflict doesn't make relationships weaker; the opposite is true. Failing is part of relationships—it's the way we come back from failure that can make us stronger.

According to findings by the Gottman Institute, what separates the healthiest couples ("master couples") from unhealthy couples ("disaster couples") is the ability to repair.[8] In other words, we will all fail in our relationships. It's inevitable, because none of us are perfect. But the way we repair, or come back from conflict, makes the difference between a healthy relationship and an unhealthy one.

Repair is a relational skill that can be developed. In doing so, we learn to communicate through tough issues and draw even closer, with a deeper, clearer understanding of the other person.

Instead of putting our energy into avoiding conflict (which ends up hurting relationships), we need to lean into our humanity. We will mess up—conflict is normal. Healthy repair is the way to build strong, lasting relationships.

• • •

No matter what your false script is—being so independent you ignore relationships or looking to a partner to meet all your needs or expecting fairy-tale, conflict-free relationships—it's time to begin breaking this unhealthy pattern.

GETTING CLOSE

Chelsea's pattern was easy to spot:

- **Stressor:** being single in her forties
- **Thought:** *I'm going to be alone forever.*
- **Emotions:** shame and fear
- **Protection:** settling too quickly and choosing guys who were fun but emotionally unavailable

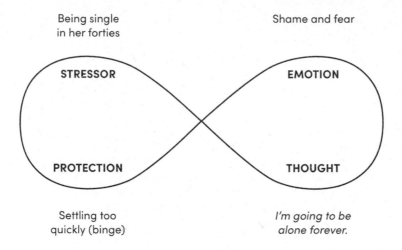

Being single
in her forties

Shame and fear

Settling too
quickly (binge)

*I'm going to be
alone forever.*

Chelsea thought the answer was to simply find the right guy who would be able to commit to her (i.e., change her circumstances). She longed for me to tell her the right thing to do, but I knew that wasn't what she needed. It was clear that her relationship with relationships was what needed to change.

The more we talked, the more obvious it became that there was a deeper, more insidious Negativity Loop at work:

- **Stressor:** someone getting close
- **Thought:** *They won't like who I really am.*
- **Emotions:** shame and fear
- **Protection:** staying guarded in healthy relationships; jumping ship for unhealthy relationships

The problem wasn't that Chelsea was attracted to "bad boys." It was that she consistently (though unconsciously) pushed away emotionally healthy guys because she feared they wouldn't like who she really was.

Chelsea's deep family wounds made her fear she wasn't lovable,

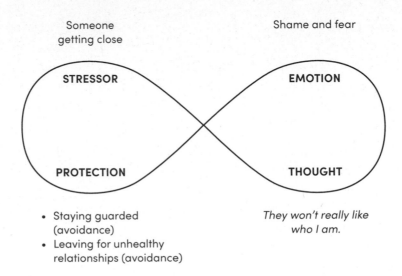

Someone
getting close

Shame and fear

STRESSOR

EMOTION

PROTECTION

THOUGHT

- Staying guarded
  (avoidance)
- Leaving for unhealthy
  relationships (avoidance)

*They won't really like
who I am.*

and her divorce fueled the shame that she was unworthy. Her false script came from her family and her church, which told her that her happiness depended on finding a romantic relationship that would lead to marriage and kids—having the perfect family. To avoid these negative emotions, she chose the wrong guys because she thought being in a relationship proved her worth. In addition, these guys felt safe to her. Their lack of emotional connection meant they wouldn't get close, which was a way to protect herself.

In our work together, Chelsea began to unpack this truth: *I am okay, just as I am.* Eventually she was able to say, *I am created in God's image. I am wonderfully made.* She practiced living into this new identity and staying emotionally present when challenging her false scripts. Then she built her self-awareness, learning what she wanted in her relationships.

She focused on gratitude for the positive relationships she already had in her life: her relationship with her mother, brothers, sisters, and plenty of friends. She created a Joyful Purpose that redefined connection in her life: "To show love to myself and all others. To invest in all forms of connection (not just romantic ones) so I can enjoy feeling loved and known by those who are important to me. To help others know they are safe and loved in my presence."

With this purpose, she was able to reap joy from all the relationships in her life, not just romantic ones. Whenever the Judge went on the attack, she practiced kind thought toward herself in response.

To build on her Joyful Purpose and to help her date more emotionally available guys, I issued Chelsea a "10 Date Challenge." The idea was simple. Her mission was to gather a group of friends and tell them that she was committing to ten dates—and having fun on those dates. These didn't have to be ten dates with ten different guys. She could go on ten dates with the same person, or if she wasn't clicking with someone, she could go out with someone else for a total of ten dates.

The goal was to give Chelsea the chance to get to know someone past the initial awkward phases while also giving her the opportunity to get to know other people. The point of involving her friends was to make it more fun and to invite them to help her see her blind spots.

We're used to keeping the dating part of our lives to ourselves. But involving people you trust in your dating life allows a unique opportunity to invest in your friendships, your community, and yourself. Even if Chelsea didn't connect with anyone romantically during the challenge, she would still benefit from stronger relationships with her friends.

Chelsea accepted the challenge, and her friends gave her wise counsel regarding the guys she dated. On date number nine, she met a man who was emotionally available and a good match for her. Now she's engaged to him.

Of course, changing your relationship to relationships doesn't guarantee your circumstances will change. But it will help you reap fruits of joy and fulfillment in the relationships you have. And as you pursue emotional health and joy, who knows what God will bring about in your life?

BREAKING PATTERNS IN MARRIAGE

The most common relationship challenges we see at Enjoyco involve marital stress. One partner may betray the other's trust, or one partner can't see the other's viewpoint, and they face compounding Negativity Loops.

If you're struggling in your marriage right now, you may be wondering, *How can I use the start-from-joy approach in my relationship?* The best way to interrupt your negative patterns may be to work with a therapist who knows your story. But here's how you can get started applying these principles in your marriage.

1. Craft your Negativity Loops.

Before you engage your partner, take some time apart to plot out all the sections in your Negativity Loop. This builds your awareness about what your triggers are and what is needed for change to occur. This also helps you focus on your half of the equation. After all, no conflict in marriage is a one-way street. Taking responsibility for your part of the conflict models to your partner what it might look like for them to take responsibility for their side. It's from this tender soil that you can grow fruitful seeds for your marriage while also strengthening the tools in your relational toolbox.

For example, in creating your own Negativity Loop, you might realize you have a protection response of withdrawing from conflict, which compounds the frustration or anger your partner is feeling.

Once you have clarity on your individual patterns, you can be aware of how they're triggered in marital conflicts. To stop your loop from sabotaging your relationship and escalating the conflict, start by identifying your emotions and the story behind them. This healthy expression of emotions provides you with the safety you need to break the loop.

2. Be curious with emotions.

If you want to break a Negativity Loop, start by owning your emotions. When relational conflict strikes, the single most important action you can take is to identify an emotion, name it, and express it to your partner so they can validate the emotion.

In order to repair after a conflict, it's important to establish emotional safety. If you and your partner spend your energy trying to escape hard emotions, the conflict perpetuates. But sometimes a single question can stop a conflict from spiraling further: "Hey, can I process something with you?" If your partner leans in, don't be afraid to own your feeling, name it, and give the story behind it.

For instance, you might say, "When you come home late, it leaves me feeling neglected and lonely. It triggers the same feelings I had when my parents came home late when I was a kid." Your partner might respond with, "I understand that. I hate feeling lonely. When you say I come home late all the time, it makes me feel shame because I don't want to be that type of parent. That's why I got defensive."

3. Interrupt your loops.

To interrupt your loops, you can take a wise action based on the type of protection response you struggle with:

- bingeing → boundaries
- avoidance → attentiveness
- rage → reconnection and repair

If you struggle with bingeing responses in your relationships, such as emotional manipulation, flooding your partner, helicopter parenting, or overjustifying when you make a mistake, the best solution is to develop boundaries. That means having a clear understanding of where you end and where someone else begins. It means owning what's yours and giving back to the other person what's theirs. Instead of holding your friends, parents, spouse, and children responsible for your emotions, you create boundaries that respect their individuality while also caring for your needs.

If you self-sabotage with avoidance responses, such as withdrawing, escaping conflict, or shutting down emotionally, the solution is to give attention to your relationships. When you feel the temptation to pull back, lean in. Instead of walking away or stonewalling your partner, express that you need to take a minute to cool down before reengaging. Your wise action is giving your relationships the attention they need to thrive.

If your relationships fall victim to rage responses, such as blaming, criticizing, or becoming defensive, the solution is to reconnect and repair. Dr. John Gottman calls the four most common rage responses "the Four Horsemen of the Apocalypse." They are criticism (attacking your partner's personality or character), contempt (showing moral superiority and reducing your partner's sense of self), defensiveness (protecting yourself from an attack by reversing the blame), and stonewalling (refusing to talk and disengaging from your partner).[9] The antidotes to these attacks include showing respect and appreciation for your partner, using gentle start-ups to tough conversations, and turning toward your partner rather than away from them.

When you're facing marital strife, take the appropriate wise action to change the trajectory of your conflicts.

4. Find your Joyful Purpose.

Conflict tends to pull us into our individual worlds. We become blind to our partner's needs and fight to have our own needs met. But it's possible to embrace a Joyful Purpose in marriage—a shared vision for the relationship. Dr. John Gottman calls this creating *shared meaning*, which leads to the most successful romantic relationships.[10]

When false scripts and Negativity Loops threaten to isolate you and your partner, you can return to your shared Joyful Purpose. For instance, if you realize you're frequently working late and leaving your partner to put the kids to bed alone, it might not be because you have a busy workload but rather because you feel guilty about a debt that's weighing on you. If your actions go against your Joyful Purpose, you can stop yourself by saying, "I don't think this matches our Joyful Purpose" or "How can we live out our values and purpose here?" These statements stop the gravitational pull of false scripts and reorient you to being a team.

5. Make it fun.

Adding fun and play into your relationship helps build positive emotional reservoirs. These reserves act as a buffer when conflict strikes.

It might sound basic, but there's actually scientific evidence that makes a case for regular date nights. The National Marriage Project at the University of Virginia did a study on the impact of date nights on marriages. They discovered that date nights lead to a higher quality of relationship by fostering greater communication, novelty, eros (passionate love), commitment, and stress relief.

Husbands and wives who have couple time (time when they're intentionally together) at least once a week enjoy at least three times more sexual satisfaction in their marriage than those who have couple time less than once a week. The same number applies to their satisfaction with communication. Husbands and wives who have couple time at least once a week are at least twice as committed to their marriage than those who have couple time less than once a week.

Here's the key to making date nights stick: commit to having out-of-the-box dates. Don't rely only on dinner and a movie—plan novel experiences from time to time. Because our brains are drawn to novelty, breaking the mold helps ensure that your time together is something you're drawn to repeat.[11]

HOW TO HEAL SHAME IN RELATIONSHIPS

Soon after I started my new job, Carly and I were sitting in a burger restaurant waiting for our food when she told me she'd written a poem about me. I stopped fiddling with my straw and paid attention. *This is the moment I've been waiting for!* Typically she writes poetry about God and the opportunity for worship in ordinary, everyday life. But now she'd written about me! *Finally,* I thought. I felt so honored.

She handed me her phone so I could read the poem. To my surprise, it wasn't a love poem. Here's what it said:

Cavern wanderer,
You carved your name into the deep dark
earth of that mountain wall
just to prove that you were here at all
just dying to be known.
Cavern wanderer,
You'll never know where life will lead you.
Boldly step on lush green grass of open land
and broad horizon. Breathe in and open
that part of you that's longing to be found.

I was stunned. The haunting beauty of her words penetrated me and made me feel understood at the same time.

"I don't know how to end it," she said.

I knew why. It was because my story wasn't over yet. I had left my business thinking that would solve my problems. But even after Myron helped me untangle my false scripts around work, there was an unresolved issue in my life: my relationships.

If shame occurs

in relationships,

it can also be healed

in relationships.

My relationships were still struggling under the weight of my shame. I pushed people away, and I didn't have deep community. Even Carly felt distant to me.

I realized that the further I wandered into that empty void, trying to fill it with something to prove I was worthy, the more distance I would create between me and the people I loved. Maybe they would get my monuments when I was gone, but they never asked for that. They wanted *me*.

Carly couldn't follow me into the cavern. She was on the outside, waiting for me to venture out and allow myself to be known.

Shame is tricky like this. It convinces us that no one wants us, that we don't deserve to be in relationships, so we push people away.

During my time with Myron, I learned something about shame: it most often strikes in the context of relationships. That's because we don't experience the whiplash of shame unless someone deals the blow. But that's actually good news. If shame occurs in relationships, it can also be healed in relationships.

After reading Carly's poem, I knew what I had to do. I needed to be willing to take a risk, come out of my cavern, and be my full self in my relationships. No more facade. No more mask. No more pretending.

As I made myself more vulnerable, allowing others to see both the messy parts and the shiny parts of me, shame slowly unclenched itself from my heart. And this wasn't just in my relationships with other people; it also happened in my relationship with God. For too long, I'd been the Prodigal Son rehearsing my answers on the way back to the Father. I thought I had to prove myself to God, but I didn't know what I had to offer. So I hid. But as I offered more of myself to God and started exploring a true personal relationship with him, he surprised me. On my journey back home to him, I found that God was already running toward me, arms wide open, ready to meet me and wash away the shame I'd held close for so long.

One of the wisest actions we can take to create joy in our lives is to open ourselves fully to our relationships. The more we hide, disconnect, and play it safe, the more power we give to shame, guilt, and fear. It's scary—I know. But as we consistently turn toward one another, we compound our joy. And this joy spreads into the crevices of our lives, making way for the greatest change to occur.

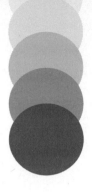

Conclusion

THE GOAL OF POSITIVE CHANGE

"I think it's time to say our goodbyes."

Myron rose from his armchair, and with a smile on his face, he gave me one last handshake. I (Neal) experienced only a few seconds of panic before I realized he was right. I knew the way forward when it came to healing my relationship with work and relationships. Now it was time for me to practice the truths I'd learned.

"Can I come back if I need to?" I asked.

"You can always come back," Myron replied.

As I walked out the door, the warm sun greeted my face and filled me with hope. I was a different person than I'd been when I first walked into Myron's office. Not only had I become aware of the patterns of shame, guilt, and fear in my life, but I had healed them. Now joy was an accessible reality.

Pulling out of the parking lot, I felt a new story beginning. I was no longer afraid of repeating the past; I was afraid of giving up on the future.

• • •

Like Neal, I (Carly) have been stuck under the influence of false scripts—around my body, my money, and my work. These areas of my life plateaued, preventing me from experiencing God's vision for them. It was only when I sought therapy and coaching that I was able to experience healing in these areas.

Maybe you're in the midst of this struggle right now. Your life has a lot of good in it, but you know something is missing. You feel it in your bones—there's a higher purpose for your body, your money, your work, your relationships, and every other area of your life. False scripts have swept in and distorted this higher purpose. You've bought into the lie that once you lose the weight, you'll finally feel the happiness you long for. Once you make more money, your life will become easy, happy, and meaningful. Once you become successful in your job, you'll be able to start living with joy. Once you find someone who loves you unconditionally, you'll live happily ever after.

But we are here to tell you: your personal happiness is not the goal of positive change; it's the by-product.

The true purpose behind positive change is to partner in what God is doing in us and through us. When we heal our emotional relationships, we get to fully participate in the active redemption plan God has set out for this world. This is what God intended for our positive change—not only that we would change, but that the world would change because of us. And as we journey on this path, our happiness and joy will compound.

• • •

To be honest, I (Neal) used to be a little frightened of joy. I thought if I allowed joy to seize me and open my eyes to all the goodness baked into the present, then I would stop striving for the future.

This is what God intended for our positive change—not only that we would change, but that the world would change because of us.

Discontentment, I believed, kept me motivated. As long as I bought into the false scripts about delaying happiness for the future, then I would keep hustling, working hard, and putting in the hours to achieve future joy. Yet all this did was burn me out.

Giving myself permission to embrace joy now, without changing anything, surprised me in all the best ways. For one thing, choosing joy didn't make me apathetic to change; rather, it pushed me to see what more could be possible. I also thought I would sacrifice a happier future if I allowed myself to experience joy today. If I was disappointed today, I thought things could only go up from here. But what I learned is that joy never peaks. The more you allow it to reverberate through your life, the stronger it becomes.

I realized that if I didn't start from joy, most of the change I was pushing for was simply about helping me feel better, not making the world better. When I released the shame, guilt, and fear associated with positive change, it became less about self-improvement and more about improving the people, community, and world around me. When I allowed for joy in the moment, it opened me up to what God is doing in the world and how I could partner with him.

The start-from-joy life is not something that occurs when all your circumstances line up. It's a choice you make for today.

It's choosing to recognize your worth outside your weight, your money, your professional accomplishments, your relationships, and anything else.

It's choosing to end the patterns that burn you out.

It's choosing to trust in a better tomorrow by allowing for more good today.

And ultimately it's choosing to align with a bigger, more fulfilling picture of positive change. It's less about us and more about what God could allow through us, if we let joy in now.

Our hope for you is that the principles in this book allow you to make a choice for joy today. While the world wants you to keep putting off joy to the future, it's possible to embrace joy as a reality that can be claimed right now. The start-from-joy life is yours for the taking.

Now go create the future with joy.

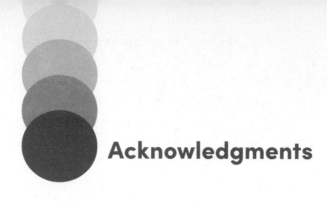

Acknowledgments

Carly and I (Neal) wrote this book in one of the most trying times of our lives. Jude had just been born, and we were overwhelmed by many life transitions hitting us at once. Yet in the midst of our uncertainty and figuring out our new life, this book was still able to enter into the world. If I ended the story there, you would think Carly and I were tough people. Who else writes a book and attends publisher meetings when their baby is just three weeks old? But the truth is, this accomplishment wouldn't have happened if it weren't for the village of support that came around us during that time.

To our literary agent, D. J. Snell: thank you for seeing the vision behind our book and getting so passionate about it. Your excitement carried us through the hard parts of getting this book out there. You were the best advocate for our book, and we can't wait to partner with you more in the future.

To Jillian, Stephanie, and the rest of the Tyndale House Publishers team: we couldn't have asked for better publishers. Thanks for taking a risk on us new authors, for getting excited about our vision, and for helping us craft a message that will change lives.

To the team at Enjoyco: if you had asked Carly and me at the beginning of 2020, when we had the idea for Enjoyco, if we could imagine it being where it is today, we would have laughed. We couldn't have imagined leading a team, not to mention having the best team of passionate people. Yet here we are. Thank you for coming alongside our bold vision and for helping people enjoy positive change. Here's to more innovation and growth for the future!

To Beth McCord, Jeff McCord, Suzie Barbour, and the rest of the Your Enneagram Coach team: when I left my job during this crazy period of transition, I didn't know what to expect. I was bracing for a difficult period of writing a book and building a business to pay our bills, all while being sleep-deprived. Then you all gave me the best opportunity I've ever had. Working with Your Enneagram Coach allowed me to keep doing what I love, write the book, and enjoy greater margin with my family. I will never be able to give back the joy you've given me. Thanks for taking a chance on me. Here's to reaching new heights together.

To Jordan Raynor: none of this would've been possible without you. Your introductions, wise counsel, and supportive presence gave birth to this book. I will never be able to repay what you've given me either. Thank you for your generous spirit and your willingness to help people like me.

To Chris Niemeyer: you've mentored me through big transitions. You've heard it all! This book is the result of your timely guidance. Thank you for pouring into my life. I'm so glad I have a model of what a good father, entrepreneur, and dreamer looks like in you.

To Donna Aufhammer: your presence has been an unexpected abundant blessing in our lives. When we were looking for a nanny to watch Jude while we wrote this book, we didn't expect to get someone who would impact our lives as much as you have. Your wisdom and joy have shaped us in a vulnerable time. We are so glad you've entered our home and brought your energy, peace, and joy with you.

And finally, thank you, God. You've always given us more than we asked for. You love showering us with abundance. May this book partner with the work you're doing and bring about positive change to a world that needs it.

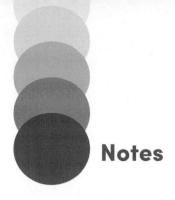

Notes

INTRODUCTION: WHAT DOES IT MEAN TO START FROM JOY?
1. Shawn Achor, *The Happiness Advantage: The Seven Principles of Positive Psychology That Fuel Success and Performance at Work* (New York: Crown Business, 2010), 3.

CHAPTER 1: THE GIFTS OF JOY
1. Chip Dodd, *The Voice of the Heart: A Call to Full Living* (Nashville: Sage Hill, 2014), 39.
2. Melanie Curtin, "Brené Brown Says This Is the Most Vulnerable Human Emotion in the World . . . and It's Not Shame," Inc.com, August 30, 2019, https://www.inc.com/melanie-curtin/brene-brown-says-this-is-most-vulnerable -human-emotion-in-world-its-not-shame.html.
3. Philippians 4:11-12.
4. Susan David, *Emotional Agility: Get Unstuck, Embrace Change, and Thrive in Work and Life* (New York: Avery Publishing, 2016), 117.
5. Dodd, *The Voice of the Heart*, 31.

CHAPTER 2: END THE MOTIVATION OF SHAME, GUILT, AND FEAR
1. Brené Brown, *The Gifts of Imperfection: Let Go of Who You Think You're Supposed to Be and Embrace Who You Are* (Center City, MN: Hazelden Publishing, 2010), 39.
2. Tanya Lewis and Ashley P. Taylor, "Human Brain: Facts, Functions, and

Anatomy," *Live Science* (updated May 28, 2021), https://www.livescience
.com/29365-human-brain.html.

3. This is often called the hedonic theory of motivation. You can learn more at
Lukasz D. Kaczmarek, "Hedonic Motivation," in *Encyclopedia of Personality
and Individual Differences*, ed. Virgil Zeigler-Hill and Todd K. Shackelford
(2017), https://doi.org/10.1007/978-3-319-28099-8_524-1.

4. Joseph Burgo, "The Risks of Joy," *Psychology Today*, September 20, 2016,
https://www.psychologytoday.com/us/blog/shame/201609/the-risks-joy.

5. Rajita Sinha et al., "Neural Activity Associated with Stress-Induced
Cocaine Craving: A Functional Magnetic Resonance Imaging Study,"
Psychopharmacology 183, no. 2 (2005): 171–80, https://doi.org/10.1007
/s00213-005-0147-8.

6. Janet Polivy and C. Peter Herman, "Dieting and Binging: A Causal Analysis,"
American Psychologist 40, no. 2 (1985): 193–201, https://doi.org/10.1037
/0003-066x.40.2.193; Stacey Colino, "Avoiding the What-the-Hell Health
Effect," *U.S. News & World Report* (November 15, 2017), https://health
.usnews.com/wellness/mind/articles/2017-11-15/avoiding-the-what-the-hell
-health-effect.

7. Matthew 25:14-30.

8. 2 Thessalonians 3:14.

9. Hosea 5:15.

10. Proverbs 14:27; 19:23.

11. Thanks to Chip Dodd for these insights in his book *The Voice of the Heart:
A Call to Full Living* (Nashville: Sage Hill, 2014).

12. Joseph Burgo, "Why Shame Is Good," *Vox*, April 18, 2019, https://www.vox
.com/first-person/2019/4/18/18308346/shame-toxic-productive.

13. Romans 10:11.

14. Dodd, *The Voice of the Heart*, 123.

15. Hebrews 10:22.

16. Adele Ahlberg Calhoun, *Spiritual Disciplines Handbook: Practices That Transform
Us* (Downers Grove, IL: InterVarsity Press, 2005), 91.

17. Psalm 111:10; Proverbs 4:7.

CHAPTER 3: BE CURIOUS WITH YOUR EMOTIONS

1. James J. Gross and Oliver P. John, "Individual Differences in Two Emotion
Regulation Processes: Implications for Affect, Relationships, and Well-Being,"
Journal of Personality and Social Psychology 85, no. 2 (August 2003): 348–62,
https://doi.org/10.1037/0022-3514.85.2.348.

2. Susan David, *Emotional Agility: Get Unstuck, Embrace Change, and Thrive in
Work and Life* (New York: Avery Publishing, 2016), 85.

3. Allyson Chiu, "Time to Ditch 'Toxic Positivity,' Experts Say: 'It's Okay Not to
Be Okay,'" *Washington Post*, August 19, 2020, http://www.washingtonpost

.com/lifestyle/wellness/toxic-positivity-mental-health-covid/2020/08/19
/5dff8d16-e0c8-11ea-8181-606e603bb1c4_story.html.
4. 1 Thessalonians 5:16-18, NLT.
5. Psalm 30:5; Proverbs 14:13.
6. John 16:20.
7. John 11:1-44.
8. Drake Baer, "How Only Being Able to Use Logic to Make Decisions Destroyed a Man's Life," *The Cut*, June 14, 2016, https://www.thecut.com/2016/06/how -only-using-logic-destroyed-a-man.html.
9. Lisa Feldman Barrett, *How Emotions Are Made: The Secret Life of the Brain* (New York: Mariner Books, 2018), 3.
10. Todd B. Kashdan, Lisa Feldman Barrett, and Patrick E. McKnight, "Unpacking Emotion Differentiation: Transforming Unpleasant Experience by Perceiving Distinctions in Negativity," *Current Directions in Psychological Science* 24, no. 1 (2015): 10–16, https://doi.org/10.1177/0963721414550708.
11. Kristin Neff, "Definition of Self-Compassion" and "The Three Elements of Self-Compassion," Self-Compassion.org, https://self-compassion.org/the-three -elements-of-self-compassion-2/.
12. Jill Bolte Taylor, "My Stroke of Insight," TED.com, February 2008, https://www.ted.com/talks/jill_bolte_taylor_my_stroke_of_insight.
13. Agnieszka Wojnarowska, Dorota Kobylinska, and Karol Lewczuk, "Acceptance as an Emotion Regulation Strategy in Experimental Psychological Research: What We Know and How We Can Improve That Knowledge," *Frontiers in Psychology* 11 (February 27, 2020): 242, https://doi.org/10.3389/fpsyg.2020 .00242.
14. Nathaniel R. Herr et al., "The Impact of Validation and Invalidation on Aggression in Individuals with Emotion Regulation Difficulties," *Personality Disorders: Theory, Research, and Treatment* 6, no. 4 (2015): 310–14, https:// doi.org/10.1037/per0000129.

CHAPTER 4: INTERRUPT YOUR LOOPS

1. Zoya Gervis, "The Average American Abandons Their New Year's Resolution by This Date," *New York Post*, January 28, 2020, https://nypost.com/2020/01/28 /the-average-american-abandons-their-new-years-resolution-by-this-date/.
2. American Psychological Association, "Lack of Willpower May Be Obstacle to Improving Personal Health and Finances," APA.org (2012), https://www.apa .org/news/press/releases/2012/02/willpower.
3. Julia K. Boehm and Sonja Lyubomirsky, "The Promise of Sustainable Happiness," *The Oxford Handbook of Positive Psychology*, 2nd ed. (Oxford University Press, 2009), 666–78, https://www.oxfordhandbooks.com/view /10.1093/oxfordhb/9780195187243.001.0001/oxfordhb-9780195187243 -e-063.

4. Ruth Davidhizar, "The Pursuit of Illness for Secondary Gain," *The Health Care Supervisor* 13, no. 1 (September 1, 1994), 10–15.
5. "Brené Brown on Blame," RSA Shorts, February 3, 2015, https://www.youtube.com/watch?v=RZWf2_2L2v8.
6. Matthew 11:29, ESV.
7. Philippians 2:6-8.

CHAPTER 5: CHALLENGE FALSE SCRIPTS

1. C. S. Lewis, *The Screwtape Letters*, in *The Complete C. S. Lewis Signature Classics* (New York: HarperOne, 2007), 220.
2. Adapted from Pia Mellody, "Five Core Areas for Healing" in Jan Bergstrom, *Gifts from a Challenging Childhood: Creating a Practice for Becoming Your Healthiest Self* (Mill Valley, CA: Mountain Stream Publishing Company, 2019), 11–12.
3. Mark 2:27; 1 Timothy 4:4.
4. Henry Cloud and John Townsend, *Safe People: How to Find Relationships That Are Good for You and Avoid Those That Aren't* (Grand Rapids, MI: Zondervan, 2016), 27.
5. Margaret Jaworski, "The Negativity Bias: Why the Bad Stuff Sticks," Psycom.net, February 19, 2020, https://www.psycom.net/negativity-bias.
6. Acts 2.
7. Aundi Kolber, *Try Softer: A Fresh Approach to Move Us out of Anxiety, Stress, and Survival Mode—and into a Life of Connection and Joy* (Carol Stream, IL: Tyndale House Publishers, 2020), 34.
8. Brad Klontz and Ted Klontz, *Mind Over Money: Overcoming the Money Disorders That Threaten Our Financial Health* (New York: Broadway Books, 2009), 211.
9. Henry Cloud and John Townsend, *Boundaries: When to Say Yes, How to Say No to Take Control of Your Life* (Grand Rapids, MI: Zondervan, 2017), 27.

CHAPTER 6: CALL OUT THE JUDGE

1. Quita Christison, "We All Make Snap Judgments about Each Other—Here's How to Stop," TED-Ed, April 20, 2020, https://blog.ed.ted.com/2020/04/20/we-all-make-snap-judgments-about-each-other-heres-how-to-stop/.
2. 1 John 4:18, NLT.
3. Atsushi Oshio and Tatiana Meshkova, "Eating Disorders, Body Image, and Dichotomous Thinking among Japanese and Russian College Women," *Health* 4, no. 7 (July 2012): 392–99, https://www.scirp.org/journal/paperinformation.aspx?paperid=21188.
4. Benoît Monin and Dale T. Miller, "Moral Credentials and the Expression of Prejudice," *Journal of Personality and Social Psychology* 81, no. 1 (2001): 33–43, https://psycnet.apa.org/record/2001-07168-003.
5. Akihiko Masuda et al., "Cognitive Defusion and Self-Relevant Negative Thoughts: Examining the Impact of a Ninety Year Old Technique," *Behaviour*

Research and Therapy 42, no. 4 (April 2004): 477–85, https://pubmed.ncbi
.nlm.nih.gov/14998740/.

6. Kristin D. Neff, Kristin L. Kirkpatrick, and Stephanie S. Rude, "Self-
Compassion and Adaptive Psychological Functioning," *Journal of Research
in Personality* 41 (2007): 139–54, https://self-compassion.org/wp-content
/uploads/publications/JRP.pdf.

7. Mark R. Leary et al., "Self-Compassion and Reactions to Unpleasant Self-
Relevant Events: The Implications of Treating Oneself Kindly," *Journal of
Personality and Social Psychology* 92, no. 5 (2007): 887–904, https://doi.org
/10.1037/0022-3514.92.5.887.

8. Galatians 5:22.

9. 2 Timothy 1:7, NKJV.

CHAPTER 7: FIND YOUR JOYFUL PURPOSE

1. Angela Duckworth, *Grit: The Power of Passion and Perseverance* (New York:
Scribner, 2016), 143.

2. Debra Trampe, Diederik A. Stapel, and Frans W. Siero, "The Self-Activation
Effect of Advertisements: Ads Can Affect Whether and How Consumers Think
about the Self," *Journal of Consumer Research* 37, no. 6 (April 2011): 1030–45,
https://www.jstor.org/stable/10.1086/657430.

3. John Piper, *Desiring God: Meditations of a Christian Hedonist* (Colorado Springs,
CO: Multnomah, 2011), 28.

4. Luke 2:41-49.

5. Luke 10:38-42.

6. Matthew 28:19-20.

7. Anna Redsand, *Viktor Frankl: A Life Worth Living* (New York: Clarion Books,
2006), 18.

8. 2 Corinthians 1:3-4.

CHAPTER 8: MAKE IT FUN

1. Greg McKeown, *Essentialism: The Disciplined Pursuit of Less* (New York:
Currency, 2014), 85.

2. Psalm 37:4.

3. Zephaniah 3:17.

4. Acts 2:42-47.

5. Boris Cheval et al., "Avoiding Sedentary Behaviors Requires More Cortical
Resources than Avoiding Physical Activity: An EEG Study," *Neuropsychologia*
119 (October 2018): 68–80, https://pubmed.ncbi.nlm.nih.gov/30056055/.

6. *University of Chicago Press Journals*, "Could Learning Self-Control Be Enjoyable?,"
Science Daily, September 21, 2010, https://www.sciencedaily.com/releases/2010
/09/100920172744.htm.

7. Kaitlin Woolley and Ayelet Fishbach, "For the Fun of It: Harnessing Immediate
Rewards to Increase Persistence in Long-Term Goals," *Journal of Consumer*

Research 42, no. 6 (2016): 952–66, https://academic.oup.com/jcr/article
-abstract/42/6/952/2358882?redirectedFrom=fulltext.

8. "Simply Fearing the Day Will Be Stressful Worsens Memory, Focus,
Productivity," StudyFinds.org, July 30, 2018, https://www.studyfinds
.org/fearing-day-stressful-worsens-memory-focus-productivity/.

9. "Self-Control: Dan Ariely at TEDxDuke," YouTube, April 18, 2011,
https://www.youtube.com/watch?v=PPQhj6ktYSo.

10. "Using 'The Hunger Games' to Encourage Healthier Choices," *Knowledge@
Wharton*, UPenn.edu, November 19, 2013, https://knowledge.wharton.upenn
.edu/article/researchers-used-hunger-games-encourage-healthier-choices/.

11. Brené Brown, *Daring Greatly* (New York: Avery, 2015), 117.

12. Nathaniel M. Lambert et al., "A Boost of Positive Affect: The Perks of Sharing
Positive Experiences," *Journal of Social and Personal Relationships* 30, no. 1
(2013): 24–43, https://journals.sagepub.com/doi/10.1177/0265407512449400.

13. James H. Fowler and Nicholas A. Christakis, "Dynamic Spread of Happiness in
a Large Social Network: Longitudinal Analysis over 20 Years in the Framingham
Heart Study," *BMJ* 337, no. a2338 (2008): 1–9, https://www.bmj.com/content
/337/bmj.a2338.

14. Shelly L. Gable, Gian C. Gonzaga, and Amy Strachman, "Will You Be There
for Me When Things Go Right? Supportive Responses to Positive Event
Disclosures," *Journal of Personality and Social Psychology* 91, no. 5 (2006):
904–17, https://doi.org/10.1037/0022-3514.91.5.904.

15. C. S. Lewis, *Letters to Malcolm: Chiefly on Prayer* (San Diego: Harvest, 1964), 93.

CHAPTER 9: ENJOY YOUR HEALTH

1. Linda Searing, "The Big Number: 45 Million Americans Go on a Diet Each
Year," *Washington Post*, January 1, 2018, https://www.washingtonpost.com
/national/health-science/the-big-number-45-million-americans-go-on-a-diet
-each-year/2017/12/29/04089aec-ebdd-11e7-b698-91d4e35920a3_story.html.

2. Christy Harrison, "What Is Diet Culture?," ChristyHarrison.com, August 10,
2018, https://christyharrison.com/blog/what-is-diet-culture.

3. "Global Weight Management Industry," ReportLinker, December 17, 2020,
GlobeNewswire.com, https://www.globenewswire.com/news-release/2020
/12/17/2147220/0/en/Global-Weight-Management-Industry.html.

4. Christy Harrison, "How to Avoid Falling for the Wellness Diet," ChristyHarrison
.com, April 9, 2018, https://christyharrison.com/blog/the-wellness-diet.

5. 1 Corinthians 6:19.

6. 1 Timothy 4:3-4.

7. John 21:1-14.

8. To learn more about the racism behind diet culture, see Sabrina Strings, *Fearing
the Black Body: The Racial Origins of Fat Phobia* (New York: NYU Press, 2019).

9. Amanda MacMillan, "Here's How to Make Yourself Love Exercise," *Time*, May 30,
2017, https://time.com/4796079/exercise-fitness-motivation/.

CHAPTER 10: ENJOY YOUR MONEY

1. Matthew 6:24.
2. Brad Klontz and Ted Klontz, *Mind over Money: Overcoming the Money Disorders That Threaten Our Financial Health* (New York: Broadway Books, 2009), 11.
3. Exodus 32:2-4.
4. 1 Timothy 6:10.
5. Brené Brown, *The Gifts of Imperfection: Let Go of Who You Think You're Supposed to Be and Embrace Who You Are* (Center City, MN: Hazelden Publishing, 2010), 10.
6. Sybil Carrère and John M. Gottman, "Predicting Divorce among Newlyweds from the First Three Minutes of a Marital Conflict Discussion," *Family Process* 38, no. 3 (September 1999): 293–301, https://doi.org/10.1111/j.1545-5300.1999.00293.x.
7. University of Texas at Austin, "Spending on Experiences versus Possessions Advances More Immediate Happiness," *Science Daily*, March 9, 2020, sciencedaily.com/releases/2020/03/200309130020.htm.
8. Ashley V. Whillans et al., "Buying Time Promotes Happiness," *Proceedings of the National Academy of Sciences of the United States of America* 114, no. 32 (July 24, 2017): 8523–27, https://www.pnas.org/content/114/32/8523.

CHAPTER 11: ENJOY YOUR WORK

1. Phillip Kane, "The Great Resignation Is Here, and It's Real," Inc.com, August 26, 2021, https://www.inc.com/phillip-kane/the-great-resignation-is-here-its-real.html.
2. Jenna Goudreau, "Find Happiness at Work," *Forbes*, March 4, 2010, https://www.forbes.com/2010/03/04/happiness-work-resilience-forbes-woman-well-being-satisfaction.html.
3. "Survey: Half of Americans Consider Themselves Modern-Day Workaholics," February 5, 2019, StudyFinds.org, https://www.studyfinds.org/survey-half-americans-consider-themselves-modern-day-workaholics/.
4. Emma Seppälä and Julia Moeller, "1 in 5 Employees Is Highly Engaged and at Risk of Burnout," *Harvard Business Review*, February 2, 2018, https://hbr.org/2018/02/1-in-5-highly-engaged-employees-is-at-risk-of-burnout.
5. Genesis 2:15.
6. Genesis 2:2-3.
7. Amy Wrzesniewski et al., "Jobs, Careers, and Callings: People's Relations to Their Work," *Journal of Research in Personality* 31, no. 1 (March 1997): 21–33, https://doi.org/10.1006/jrpe.1997.2162.

CHAPTER 12: ENJOY YOUR RELATIONSHIPS

1. Romans 1:6.
2. Roy F. Baumeister and Mark R. Leary, "The Need to Belong: Desire for Interpersonal Attachments as a Fundamental Human Motivation," *Psychological*

Bulletin 117, no. 3 (June 1995): 497–529, https://doi.org/10.1037/0033-2909 .117.3.497.

3. Shimon Saphire-Bernstein and Shelley E. Taylor, "Close Relationships and Happiness," *Oxford Handbook of Happiness* (Oxford, UK: Oxford University Press, 2013), https://www.oxfordhandbooks.com/view/10.1093/oxfordhb /9780199557257.001.0001/oxfordhb-9780199557257-e-060.

4. Vivek Murthy, "Work and the Loneliness Epidemic," *Harvard Business Review*, September 26, 2017, https://hbr.org/2017/09/work-and-the-loneliness-epidemic.

5. Sue Johnson, *Love Sense: The Revolutionary New Science of Romantic Relationships* (New York: Little, Brown and Company, 2013), 22.

6. Genesis 2:18.

7. Isaiah 43:1-7.

8. Kyle Benson, "Repair Is the Secret Weapon of Emotionally Connected Couples," The Gottman Institute, February 23, 2017, https://www.gottman.com/blog /repair-secret-weapon-emotionally-connected-couples/.

9. John M. Gottman and Nan Silver, *The Seven Principles for Making Marriage Work* (New York: Harmony Books, 2015), 32–39.

10. Gottman and Silver, *The Seven Principles for Making Marriage Work*, 28.

11. W. Bradford Wilcox and Jeffrey Dew, "The Date Night Opportunity," The National Marriage Project, 2012, http://nationalmarriageproject.org/wp -content/uploads/2012/05/NMP-DateNight.pdf.

About the Authors

Neal Samudre is the cofounder and CEO of Enjoyco, an emotional health and wellness company designed to help individuals enjoy positive change. He is also a former marketing executive, where his leadership helped several Inc. 5000 companies scale. Neal is a viral writer on the subject of joy and positive psychology. More than five million people have shared his articles, and more than 500,000 people have completed his devotionals on the Bible App. Neal has been featured at the Catalyst Conference and in national publications such as *Relevant* magazine, *Church Leaders* magazine, *Huffington Post*, and more. He lives with his wife, Carly, and son, Jude, outside Nashville.

Carly Samudre, LPC-MHSP, is a licensed professional counselor in the greater Nashville area. She is also the cofounder of Enjoyco, an emotional health and wellness company that helps individuals enjoy positive change. In addition to her therapy practice, she is a sought-after speaker for women's ministries, leading women at all stages of their faith into deeper discipleship and biblical understanding. Carly holds a master's degree in clinical mental health counseling from Gordon-Conwell Theological Seminary. She lives outside of Nashville with her husband, Neal, and their son, Jude.

Your successful, positive, and more joyful life starts now.

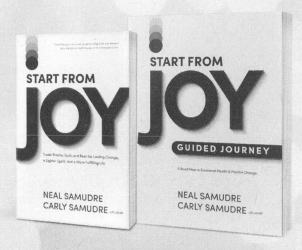

With *Start from Joy* and the *Start from Joy Guided Journey*, you'll:

- discover how you can use the gifts of joy to stick with positive change,
- develop a clearer picture of why your emotional patterns hold you back and how you can start making your emotions work for you, and
- heal your relationship with your body, work, money, and other people through easy, practical action steps.

Leave shame, guilt, and fear behind and create the fulfilling life you were always meant to live!

www.enjoyco.com

CP1793

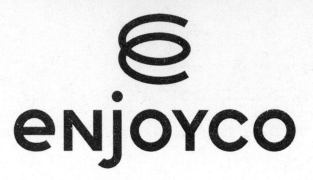

Get the Tools to Change Your Life

At Enjoyco, we believe positive change should be a clear and enjoyable experience. Through our tools and teachings, we simplify emotional health and wellness so you can create lasting change.

If you loved the tools we mentioned in the book, get access to them and more at . . .

enjoycowellness.com/sfj